D0401964

Conversations on Dying

Advance Praise for *Conversations on Dying*

It might surprise you to discover that a book about death could be so brimming with life. A beautifully hopeful story of love, family, and friendship and an undeniable argument for compassion at the end of life.

— Charlotte Gill, author of *Ladykiller*

It seems strange to call this book rejuvenating, since it peers so intently at mortality, but *Conversations on Dying* is just that. It reminds us that death is as natural a part of life as birth, and craves our thoughtful attention. The wisdom contained in these pages is irrefutable, and urges a candid approach to death that eases suffering for the person leaving, and for the loved ones left behind.

— Kristen den Hartog, author of *And Me Among Them* and *The Occupied Garden*

Phil Dwyer guides us through the death of Dr. Larry Librach and infuses new colour and life into issues of patient-centric care and palliative medicine. Both Dwyer and Librach show tremendous courage and generosity throughout the book, inviting us to witness their vulnerability and pain in their own examinations of mortality. Dwyer's narration is equal parts poetic and practical, using the energy of storytelling to offer concrete direction to patients, family members, and providers facing life-and-death decisions in contemporary healthcare.

— Julie Devaney, author of *My Leaky Body*

Conversations on dying

A PALLIATIVE-CARE PIONEER FACES HIS OWN DEATH

Phil Dwyer

DUNDURN
TORONTO

Copyright © Phil Dwyer, 2016

All rights reserved. No part of this publication may be reproduced, stored in a retrieval system, or transmitted in any form or by any means, electronic, mechanical, photocopying, recording, or otherwise (except for brief passages for purposes of review) without the prior permission of Dundurn Press. Permission to photocopy should be requested from Access Copyright.

Editor: Cheryl Hawley
Design: Courtney Horner
Cover Design: Sarah Beaudin
Printer: Webcom

Library and Archives Canada Cataloguing in Publication

Dwyer, Phil, 1955-, author
Conversations on dying : a palliative-care pioneer faces his own death / Phil Dwyer.

Includes bibliographical references.
Issued in print and electronic formats.
ISBN 978-1-4597-3193-6 (paperback).--ISBN 978-1-4597-3194-3 (pdf).--
ISBN 978-1-4597-3195-0 (epub)

1. Librach, Larry--Death and burial. 2. Pancreas--Cancer--Patients--Death. 3. Pancreas--Cancer--Palliative treatment. 4. Death--Psychological aspects. 5. Terminal care. I. Title.

R726.8.D89 2016 155.9'37 C2015-908154-8
C2015-908155-6

1 2 3 4 5 20 19 18 17 16

Conseil des Arts du Canada
Canada Council for the Arts

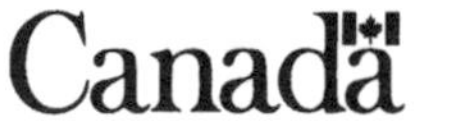

ONTARIO ARTS COUNCIL
CONSEIL DES ARTS DE L'ONTARIO
an Ontario government agency
un organisme du gouvernement de l'Ontario

We acknowledge the support of the **Canada Council for the Arts** and the **Ontario Arts Council** for our publishing program. We also acknowledge the financial support of the **Government of Canada** through the **Canada Book Fund** and **Livres Canada Books**, and the **Government of Ontario** through the **Ontario Book Publishing Tax Credit** and the **Ontario Media Development Corporation**.

Care has been taken to trace the ownership of copyright material used in this book. The author and the publisher welcome any information enabling them to rectify any references or credits in subsequent editions.

— J. Kirk Howard, President

The publisher is not responsible for websites or their content unless they are owned by the publisher.

Printed and bound in Canada.

VISIT US AT

Dundurn.com | @dundurnpress | Facebook.com/dundurnpress | Pinterest.com/dundurnpress

Dundurn
3 Church Street, Suite 500
Toronto, Ontario, Canada
M5E 1M2

For Larry, who never wavered, never flinched,
and John, my gateway to the world's wonder

CONTENTS

CHAPTER 1

Proposal

In the lobby bar of Toronto's Delta Chelsea, a girl sits at the bar nursing a dirty martini. I'm not even on her radar. My skinny jeans and Blundstone boots put me in the wrong demographic. She's tuned in to suits and neckties, the accoutrements of a company AmEx. Which is fine by me. I'm waiting for someone else entirely. I choose an armchair in the middle of the bar, facing the hotel lobby, the more easily to see and be seen.

It's March 2013, and a light snow is falling outside. So when I spot a man in a forest-green-and-navy anorak tack toward the bar, make a quick pass, and tack away again, I stand and call: "Larry." He turns, holds his hand up to show he's spotted me amongst the late-afternoon drinkers, and bustles in. Just as Pig Pen in the *Peanuts* comic strip is always followed by a cloud of dust, Larry seems to trail a continuous cloud of energy.

If you had to imagine an archetypal favourite uncle, you'd probably come up with someone like Larry. His eyes crinkle because a smile is his face's default setting. His trademark moustache, which has been grey since I first knew him, is always neatly groomed, but it's constantly being worked — curling upward at each end. He still has a full head of hair, despite his sixty-six years, and it always gives the impression that it's on the cusp of being unruly — that it might any second explode into an Einsteinian mop.

The first time I met him, six years ago, Larry was on a health kick, which kept his weight in check to some extent. But it doesn't look like he's been to the gym in a while. His sweet tooth has taken a toll on his waistline, but it seems somehow appropriate. Svelte wouldn't suit him.

I shake his hand, still cold from the chill air outside, and gesture to the seat opposite. "Drink?"

He freezes theatrically for a second as he shrugs off his coat, his cheeks still rosy from the outside air. "Of course. Why do you think I came?" His grin still has something schoolboyish in it, an ineffable filament of the child in the man. You're never far from a wisecrack when you're with Larry.

As I sit, I gesture to the barman. He wanders over, plops a couple of paper coasters on the glass table between Larry and me. "Drink, gentlemen?"

"Do you have any single malts?" Larry says. The barman lists them. Larry chooses a ten-year-old Talisker, a full-bodied, smoky whisky. Bold and, to many people's tastes, altogether too peaty. "Bombay and tonic for me," I say.

"Now," Larry leans forward, out of the over-plush, over-upholstered embrace of the armchair, so typical of hotel bars. "How can I help?"

"Here's the idea: I want to spend a couple of months riding along with palliative-care physicians who do home visits."

"To what end?"

A fair question. I have all the data points at my command, but there's no point regurgitating them to Larry; he knows them better than I do. Hell, he was probably instrumental in creating them.

The way to hook Larry is to intrigue him, tell him something he doesn't already know. He reads so widely he knows a lot.

"Did you know researchers have been MRIing people's minds as they read?"

He leans a little further in.

"Let's say you're reading a breakfast scene. If the passage just describes the meal, what it consists of, nothing much happens. But if the scene describes the smell of the coffee, the taste of the bacon, the particular sound of the eggs frying, the parts of the brain responsible for sensing taste and smell light up."

"So it's like the reader's really experiencing the breakfast?"

"Exactly."

"Where was this published?" It's a typical Larry question. Check your sources. Find out more.

"*Poets and Writers*. Don't worry, it was based on kosher research. I'll send you the link."

"So the point is ..."

"Simply telling people that dying at home is hugely different to dying in a hospital bed isn't enough. But if you show them ..."

"It's far more powerful." He nods deeply now, persuaded by the right slug of data.

"So what's the problem?"

He knows there has to be one. My wife, Natalie, works for the Temmy Latner Centre for Palliative Care, the largest concentration of palliative-care physicians in one centre in North America, perhaps the largest in the world. Larry co-founded the Centre and, until he retired two years ago, was its director — and my wife's boss.

"You've spoken to Russell, I assume?"

Dr. Russell Goldman is Larry's successor as the Centre's director — and my wife's new boss.

"Of course. I wrote to him to explain the idea."

"And?"

"He put it to the Leadership Team."

As soon as I'd heard that, I'd known the idea was doomed. The more people involved in a decision, the more risk averse they become.

"They nixed it: a combination of concerns over patient privacy and what feels to me like paranoia over the issue of physician-assisted death, from what I gather."

From what, to be more accurate, Natalie had been able to gather. She was locked out of the room when the discussion took place: "conflict of interest," Russell said.

Physician-assisted death is already a hot topic in 2013, and only going to get more feverish in the coming few years. Palliative-care physicians have to walk a nervous and diplomatic path between two parties that are increasingly entrenched: the pro-lifers, and the pro-choicers. In this, it's very similar to debates about abortion, except here we're not talking about a fetus, we're talking about a sentient human being. One who can argue with us about their right to die.

I moped around our condo for a day or two after Russell's rejection. Finally, Natalie said: "You still really want to do this story, don't you?"

"I still think it's important, which comes to the same thing."

"Then ask Larry. If anyone can help, he can."

I wrote to him that evening. He'd taken on two new jobs since his "retirement," so I didn't expect to hear back for a few days, but it took him less than half an hour to respond.

Larry picks up his drink, takes a sip, and holds the squat tumbler between his hands. "It's almost impossible to get any hospital to agree to media requests these days," he says. "Patient privacy has everyone rattled." He takes another sip and puts the glass back down. "It's a question of knowing your way around the system. I know a few people you can speak to. Let me ask you this though: why this story?"

Why indeed? Dying and death aren't exactly popular subjects, as I've observed many times at parties when people ask Natalie what she does. "I work in palliative care" is pretty much guaranteed to kill all further conversation. It's right up there with "actually, I'm a serial killer" or "I sell insurance." And what I'm proposing is bound to stir up some uncomfortable memories for me too.

It has been a little under three years since my eldest brother died of cancer, but the memory is still raw, and I have no illusions that this story would be cathartic.

"John," I say.

Larry coached us through John's final few weeks. He'd been more incensed than me at the mismanagement of his case. "How will this help John?"

"It won't, of course. Maybe it's my way of making sense of what he went through, making something positive come out of it. Maybe it's just my way of memorializing him. But maybe we could do something that would help promote change."

He nods, smiles, and gestures toward the messenger bag at my feet. "Get your notebook out then. You'll need to take notes."

Three weeks later Natalie and I were on vacation in the tiny Caribbean island of Bequia. It was the morning of our third day. The sun flooded through the wooden blinds of our room, painting it with bright diagonal strips of sunlight. Like most Caribbean islands, Bequia has a mosquito problem, so we both lay under a mosquito net.

Natalie reached for her iPhone to check her email. I was barely awake, but a sudden intake of breath and the movement of her hand to her mouth brought me out of my sleepy daze. I raised myself onto my elbow. Her eyes welled. Distress was written all over her face as she tried to hold back the tears. I knew, whatever it was, she'd tell me when she was ready.

My mind went naturally to her mother, her sister, and her brother-in-law. They'd all had health scares in the previous few years.

"It's Larry," she said. "He's got advanced pancreatic cancer. He's been given a couple of months to live." All I could see when I closed my eyes was Larry, in that forest-green anorak of his, reaching out his hand for me to shake. Unaccountably, I was angry.

"How could he not have known?" I asked. "If it's so advanced, surely there would have been signs. Weight loss. Pain. Something?"

She pulled away a little, reached behind her for the box of tissues on the bedside table. "There may not have been any. Not with this kind of cancer. Often there are no symptoms until it's too late."

I wasn't about to argue with her. She used to work for the Canadian Cancer Society. Her father died of non-Hodgkin's lymphoma. She knows cancer.

"So there's nothing they can do?" I asked.

She shook her head. "He'll be palliative.* One of the doctors at the Centre will look after him. Probably Russell." She blew her nose, dried her eyes. "I knew something was up."

"What are you talking about? How?"

"Don't you remember? I saw them at the hospital, Larry and Faye, shortly after you met with him. I bumped into them in the lobby — they were getting off the elevator. They both seemed down. Don't you remember me telling you?"

Faye was Larry's wife. I didn't remember the conversation. I fell back onto the pillow, stared at the ceiling. The flimsy gauze of the mosquito net moved ever so gently in the trade winds that blow steadily from

---

* Although the term *palliative* is not a medical condition, it's frequently used by nurses, support workers, and physicians working in palliative care. The use of the term does not imply there is nothing more to be done for the patient. A lot can be done for them with a palliative-care approach — which is very active care.

Barbados, a hundred miles to the east. I listened to the waves breaking on the beach in Friendship Bay, at the bottom of the rise. Earlier in the week I had found it soothing.

Inevitably, Larry's news intruded itself into the simplest of pleasures — a walk along the beach, a late-afternoon Hairoun beer at the Whaleboner bar — along with the guilt of having forgotten, even for a second.

That evening we decided to have dinner close to home. There's a fancy hotel on the beach at the bottom of the hill. It's the largest hotel on the island, and the restaurant serves fresh lobster caught by local fishermen every day.

We asked for a table facing the beach. In the darkness beyond the hotel's lights, the Atlantic rolled onto the sand. It sounded mere feet away.

We chatted about our day, our plans for tomorrow, but it felt as if we were circling the big topic.

"I can't stop thinking about Larry," Natalie said.

"I know." I folded my hands around the base of my wine glass and stared down into it.

"You know, he wouldn't want us moping around our whole holiday. He'd tell us to savour it, make the most of it. He'd remind us we're fit and healthy."

I looked up, took her hand. "So that's a deal then? No moping around?" I lifted my wine glass, and she brought hers up to meet it.

"No moping," she agreed.

We drained the last drop of pleasure out of those two weeks.

When we returned to Toronto in mid-April, the first thing Natalie did when she got back to the office was get herself up to speed on Larry. He wasn't doing so well. He had a bad case of jaundice — a side effect of his tumour — and unless it could be brought under control, the couple of months he'd been given would be down to a few weeks.

Everyone was busy while we were away. Hospice Palliative Care Ontario arranged a tribute lunch for Larry and his family, to take place on April 29, a Monday. The Centre itself planned its own tribute at the end of May.

A week or so later the Centre rethought its plans and brought its tribute forward to May 2.

It was held at the home of one of the Centre's physicians — one of Larry's oldest friends, and the palliative-care doctor who'd taken on Larry's case, David Kendal. The house is an elegant old Edwardian in the leafy streets a little north of Casa Loma: the kind of Toronto neighbourhood in which it's possible to forget you're mere kilometres from the downtown of Canada's biggest city.

When we arrived, the living room already buzzed with conversation. Larry sat in a corner, dapper in a crisp white button-down, a sharp crease to his navy trousers. He was an impressive shade of yellow, and his hands were clasped over the head of a cane. The cane was new.

A line of people waited to catch a few words with him. We dove in during a brief lull. "How are you feeling?" I said. Stupidity seems to be standard issue in these awkward social moments.

"Great." He smiled, nodded toward my wine glass. "You know, that single malt I had with you was the last drink I had."

"Really? Good job it was a good one." Which it was. It cost twice as much as my gin.

"I've decided to keep a journal. I'm learning a lot about the system now I'm seeing it from the other side." He said he was also getting first-hand confirmation of what he's always maintained: the bowels are one of the most important contributors to human happiness. "I've learned what it's like to be constipated for seven days straight." Larry was known in certain palliative-care circles as the King of Constipation. I resisted the urge to ask him if he planned to abdicate his throne.

I gestured toward a knot of his former colleagues, who began to spill through the French doors at the back of the room and on to the terrace. "How are they coping with this? I imagine they're more used to this situation than I am."

"It's quite surprising. They're as lost as everyone else. They don't know how to react, what to say. Other than the customary 'Sorry.'" His voice dropped a notch. I leant in. "It's the younger ones who have the most trouble. They can cope when it's a patient, but when it's someone they know ..." He shrugged. By now another small queue had formed behind us, so we moved on.

Later in the evening everyone moved out onto the terrace, where Larry held court for a while at one of the round cast-metal patio tables. At that certain indefinable moment — late enough that everyone should have turned up, but early enough that nobody had left yet — Russell stepped forward, tapped his wine glass twice with a knife to get everyone's attention. "Now," he said, "would be a good time to say something, if anyone had anything prepared."

The first tributes were from former colleagues, most of them palliative-care physicians. They deal with death and the dying every day of their working lives. And yet some had to pause to compose themselves before they could go on. Others rendered speechless, simply stopped mid-sentence.

The most eloquent tribute came from Larry's ten-year-old granddaughter, Ella. She sat on the corner of the terrace, and remained seated, her hands folded on her lap, as she delivered her thoughts. Fearless like most children, she looked directly at her grandfather almost the entire time she was speaking. She told him he was the smartest person she knew, that she loved him, and that she'd miss him.

The second most poised speech came from Larry. After another glowing tribute came to an end he mumbled "Okay," grabbed his walking cane, and launched himself up off his chair. Despite his weakness, there was something decisive in the cast of his shoulders and the way he held his head as he struggled to stand. Time to bring the glowing tributes to an end before they descended into pathos. Loving hands helped him climb down the three stone steps from the terrace to the lawn that skirts the swimming pool. A small group of guests moved aside to accommodate him. Those of us on the terrace, the majority, looked down on him as if he were in an amphitheatre.

He thanked his friends and colleagues, mentioned one or two by name. He'd known some of them for thirty years or more. His voice never faltered, or cracked, but the hand holding the cane trembled. Another symptom, but not of cancer. A week or so before he was diagnosed with cancer his doctor confirmed Larry's own suspicions. He had early onset Parkinson's.

These men and women had helped him turn a vision — a mere idea — into a world-leading palliative-care centre. This ordinary suburban garden was brimful of people Larry mentored and inspired. Their love for him was palpable. Quiet and attentive, every so often one or another of them wiped a tear away.

What was also palpable was that what Larry built isn't just a building, a facility, a centre: it is something that lives in the hearts and minds of these doctors. It will be passed to a new generation of physicians. Larry was the pebble, these the first concentric waves.

Still there was something a little off, a little uncomfortable about the event too. This tribute was originally conceived as a retirement party to celebrate Larry's achievements. In the event it was more like a wake, with the subject in attendance, and it was unsettling.

Larry spent his entire career counselling his patients and their extended families on open communications around death. He seemed perfectly at ease. I thought I was comfortable with this enlightened approach to death too, but perhaps my cultural conditioning was stronger than I realized.

I could feel the tension in my neck and shoulders, a tightness that grew to a dull ache as the evening wore on. It was a relief when the first guests started to drift away, and we could leave. The party hadn't fully wound down. We helped one of Natalie's colleagues load the portrait of Larry that the Centre had framed as a tribute into the back of her SUV. It would be hung in the Latner Centre's entrance hall. We went back into the house to say our goodbyes, dug our bags out of the pile in the front reception room where we left them, linked hands, and started to stroll south. I took a deep breath and let it out slowly as we walked away. I could already feel the tension flowing out of my neck and shoulders.

We had no particular plan to walk all the way home, a few kilometres away. But there was something almost hypnotic about the leafy avenues of this neighbourhood that enticed us.

I relaxed a little, but there was still a vague discomfort at work, the mental equivalent of a burr trapped under clothing. As we walked we talked about Larry, both of us shocked at his rapid decline, but not surprised that he still oozed Larryness. Almost without noticing, we were home.

Over the next few days the mental burr refused to go away. There was a story here, perhaps a better one than the one I set out to tell in the first place. I'd wanted patient stories. Here was the mother of all patient stories. All I had to do was reach out.

Nothing is that simple. There was Faye and Larry's family to consider. They had precious little time left as it was. How could I intrude upon that?

I wrote him an email, sat on it for a few days, and then deleted it unsent. I wrote another, two days later. I wrote and rewrote, until I was sick of the words on the screen. I showed it to Natalie. She suggested a few changes, some subtle, some not. The email sat on my screen all day. I worked around it. It was up there, glowing through the gathering dark, when we got home from dinner that evening. I was still undecided about it. What were my motives? Larry's questions from the Delta Chelsea haunted me. "Why this story? Why now?"

Natalie cut through the indecision: "Just send it. Larry can always say no. He'll talk it over with Faye. If he doesn't want to do it he won't."

I had a hollow feeling in the pit of my stomach as I dragged the cursor to the little envelope logo at the top left of the screen, an instinct, strangely, to look away. I half expected him to be angry at this intrusion. A yes would, in some ways, be surprising. But, in the end I had to ask.

Larry took four days to respond. He wrote back to say I should call "his social secretary," and Faye would set up a time when we could meet.

CHAPTER 2

Origins

Exactly a week after my meeting with Larry in the Delta Chelsea it was the first day of Passover. That evening Larry's condo was full of the bustle and hum of guests, some friends but mostly family, gathered for the Passover Seder (the ritual feast that takes place at the beginning of Passover). The apartment was infused with the smell of tzimmes, a carrot-based meat stew that had simmered on the stove since the previous evening. The dominant sound was laughter: Larry's deep-throated chuckle mixing with the children's brighter tones.

Larry always wanted to be a doctor. I was skeptical when he told me this. *Always* stretches back to our first memories. Before we're fully aware of the options open to us. "Surely there was a time when you wanted to be a hockey player. Or a police officer, or fire fighter?"

"No. I used to play cowboys and Indians with the other kids in the neighbourhood, but I was always the cowboy doctor. Any kids in our neighbourhood who needed medical attention for cuts or grazes knew where to come. They'd come to me and I'd fix them up." I asked him how old he would have been at the time he first knew he would be a doctor. "Oh, four or five, probably."

The cowboy doctor grew up in Toronto, both his parents committed communists. Social responsibility was always important to him, which he believed was one factor in his childhood determination to practise medicine. Another was the common immigrant's mantra. "As far as our parents were concerned we could be one of four things: a doctor, a dentist, a lawyer, or an accountant." There was never any question in his mind that his destiny was doctor.

He wasn't a religious man. For him Jewish holy days like Passover were about family, community, shared values, a common history. And food. Larry loved his food. The Seder was one of his favourite events in the Jewish calendar. A time when he could enjoy his three grandchildren, and gather his friends around him.

The condo was comfortable but modest. Unostentatious, it reflected Larry's passions: the Inuit sculptures displayed on the glass shelves and the colourful original paintings on the walls spoke of thoughtful acquisitions, as did the furnishings. Careful purchases made not to impress, but because they were loved. The first time I visited I noticed an entire wall was covered with framed awards. I asked him to talk me through them. When he was finished I commented that it was an impressive display. He smiled. "We don't have space for all of them," he said. "The rest are in our locker downstairs."

When, in 2007, Natalie first announced she was going to leave her job at the Canadian Cancer Society to work with Larry at the Latner Centre, friends and colleagues said, in hushed tones, "You're going to work with Larry Librach?"

Larry spent the last thirty-five years of his career helping the dying. He was a pioneer of palliative care in Canada. If Balfour Mount is the father of palliative care in Canada (it was he who coined the term *palliative care*) then Larry was its godfather. When you review the list of his publications, appointments, awards, and achievements, Natalie's colleagues' awe is understandable. Larry's renown stretched far beyond Canada's shores. He was one of Canada's most energetic and enthusiastic advocates of end-of-life care. He helped develop the field into a speciality with uniform standards and practices.

I asked him how he got into palliative care. He worked this field when it was still considered voodoo medicine by some members of the medical establishment. He worked it when most oncologists refused to refer patients to palliative-care programs, in part because it was an admission of their own failure. It was hardly a fashionable, popular choice.

He was surprised he'd never told me the story. "In my early years of family practice, [I was in] charge of family medicine on the ward and having people die. We had forty to fifty patients to look after, and people were dying very badly, and I was ignoring them. We'd say, 'Oh, let's not see Mr. Jones, he has lung cancer and he's dying.' And the residents would ask, 'Oh, how's he's doing? Oh ya, well that's fine, let's not look at him.' I realized I was afraid to manoeuvre through the dying."

That feeling, a general feeling of unease at his discomfort with the dying, set the backdrop, but it was one case in particular that tipped the scales for Larry. "There was a twenty-eight-year-old man who I looked after in my family practice. He came to see me just before his wedding, having had some blood in his urine. I told him he should be investigated and he said, 'I'm getting married next week and I'm going off, but when I get back I'll talk to you.' He didn't tell me he was getting back in six months. So by the time he got back and he arrived in the office he was a mess. He'd lost weight, it was obvious something was going on.

"It turned out he had a cancer of his prostate which was very malignant. They biopsied him, and he almost died of a hemorrhage. He was in the critical-care unit. At that time if you were the family doctor you were left in the dark about any of your patients with cancer. You referred them to Princess Margaret or wherever, and they were looked after and spit out again. So I didn't see him again for almost … I think it was about four to five months.

"I was in the office on a Friday afternoon, in a really busy clinic, this was when I was in private practice, and his wife called me saying he'd just been sent home from the hospital and was crying out in pain and could I see him on a home visit? I thought, I've got twenty people in this office, but this guy lived maybe five minutes from the office; should I go or not? So I said okay … she sounded so desperate. I'll go over quickly. I'll take a vial of demerol or morphine or something and I'll go see him. Well, when I saw him I was totally shocked. He'd been a young, vigorous man. He looked like a concentration camp survivor with lumps all over him. Totally bald, crying out in absolute agony. They had fractured his neck on the way home in the ambulance, because he had multiple bony metastases. So I gave him a shot of demerol, called the hospital, and said, 'I'm sending him back!' And I sent him back.

"Six weeks later to the day, it was another Friday afternoon, I got the same call from his wife saying they've sent him home. 'He's got a clinic appointment in two weeks but he's still in agony. Can you come over and do something?' I arrived to find this man crying. He had one of those surgical halos on, where they put screws in your head and it sits on your shoulders to stabilize your neck. He was in absolute agony. He hadn't received pain medication for a number of days because his doctors thought he was becoming an addict. I had some morphine, so I gave him ten milligrams, but it wasn't helping him. He was clutching the piece of paper with his clinic appointment on it. I hesitantly drew up another ampule of morphine and was just about to give it to him when he died."

I was struck by how visceral Larry's memory of this still was, even after nearly forty years. This wasn't just one of his stories, a mere anecdote, chosen to make a point. As he'd told me the story his face had twisted and he'd strangled his voice in an attempt to emulate his patient's pain. I wondered if he'd noticed how often he'd used the word *agony* to describe it.

The episode was clearly seared into Larry's consciousness. It seems significant, at least in his own account of that incident, that his focus was on his patient's pain, and his own feelings of helplessness as he tried, and failed, to control it. This incident would shape the rest of Larry's career. Why else would he have been known as "The Pain Doctor"? Why else would his major publication be the hundred-and-twenty-page, spiral-bound *Pain Manual*, still the go-to resource for pain management for physicians?

"I don't know how I made it to the office. I had to go back to get a death certificate and I filled it out. That was the Friday. I went home and had a long drink, talked about it with Faye because we always talked about those things. Then on the Monday I was going to the Ontario College of Family Physicians' Annual Scientific Assembly and the first speaker was Dr. Balfour Mount. The first thing he said was that nobody has to die in pain. That was my epiphany. That was … you know, the clouds opened up, the light shone down, and I knew that was what I wanted to do. But I didn't know what it was. And then [Dr. Mount] used the term he'd coined: *palliative care*.

"I had no idea what it was. I knew there was a committee at the hospital looking at palliative care and a colleague was on the committee. They'd been meeting for two years and talking about what to do with the dying. That was when I started to get involved with the committee and then took over the committee and said 'enough of this talking, let's do something.' So we did something and got amazing support from the hospital. We got a full-time nurse, a full-time social worker, and a full-time chaplain, which was unheard of at the time for anybody in the hospital to get in a new team that quickly. It was in the days when there was a little more money around, of course."

This made perfect sense to me. I'd seen Larry at work myself. If he thought something needed doing, he did it, and worried about the consequences later. It's an attitude and an approach I've seen many times, but mostly amongst entrepreneurs and business people involved in start-ups. Before I met Larry I'd never seen it in a medical doctor.

"So why do you think that happened? Did things start moving just because you were pushing hard?"

"Yeah. We had some data which showed the same as Elizabeth Kübler-Ross's showed."

Kübler-Ross's seminal work *On Death and Dying* introduced the world to the five stages of grief: denial, anger, bargaining, depression, and acceptance. This may work for patients and their caregivers, but it didn't seem so relevant to physicians, who seemed to have a single stage: denial. "When you asked physicians whether there were any dying patients on their wards, they said no. We looked at the charts. There were nine hundred patients at Western at that time and we found two hundred people who were legitimately dying — who would die within the next year or two for sure. Many of them with cancer, many with other illnesses.

"I got into it literally by the seat of my pants. There were no guidelines. There was Kübler-Ross's book, which introduced the five stages of grief, and that was fine, but it wasn't the entire thing. The only book on pain control was the Royal Victoria Hospital manual that Bal Mount and his colleagues had written. That was a big fat mimeographed book, it wasn't published. It was handed around amongst us all. But there was really nothing much else and there were very few other people in Toronto who were doing this."

The physicians in this new field worked in isolated little pockets. So isolated from each other that it took a trip to Montreal to connect them. "I had to go to the second meeting of the International Congress in Montreal in 1978 to meet people from Toronto who were doing palliative care.

"So we learned from each other and that was one of the reasons for getting the first group together — the palliative-care work group of Toronto:

so we could sit together and share what little knowledge we had. And we had" — he paused for a fraction of a second, drew out the next word as if it had twenty *e*'s between the *l* and the *t* — "leeeeeeettle knowledge. To this day some of that knowledge has persisted without ever being questioned until I started to question my colleagues around a number of things, particularly around opioids." Opioids are drugs, like morphine, based on the pharmacology of the opium poppy.

"It almost became like a religion for some people. A lot of the people who were in it initially were driven there by their own experiences, their family experiences. They flamed out early on because you can't put that much of yourself into it. You have to have a certain amount of empathy, but you can't live for the patients. So that was a big problem."

When I'd worked with Larry several years previously I had asked all the physicians at the Latner Centre what inspired them to get into palliative care. A significant number said they'd come to palliative care through Larry — he'd spoken at a conference, or they'd met him on a committee — and had been inspired by his work and his vision.

"My attitude was always damn the torpedoes, we need to serve the people, and the only way we can do that is if we get physicians involved. It's great to have nurses involved and they need to be involved, but if physicians aren't involved it ain't gonna happen.

"We started things, and were advocates, and were willing to take the risk. There are three hundred people who identify themselves as palliative-care physicians in Canada. But some are very part-time. What you saw around the tables at my retirement party at David Kendal's house was a group of people committing themselves full-time, or major part-time, to palliative care and loving it, as difficult as it is."

One of Larry's key achievements, one that was important to him, was pioneering the use of drug pumps in patient's homes. The majority of his patients wanted to die at home, surrounded by their own possessions, being cared for by their loved ones. In our homes we are our true selves. All the artifices we prepare to shield ourselves out there in the world are stripped away. In our homes we are in control, we make the rules, we determine who passes our threshold. Home is refuge, haven, peace. It's where we create the best memories of our lives.

On the evening of the Seder, Larry was creating one such memory.

Fitting twenty-two guests around the table that divided the lounge in half was a bit of a squeeze, but it was cheerfully managed by rearranging the furniture. The armchairs in the TV corner were moved aside. The coffee table in front of the picture window that looks out over the trees and the entry to Cedarvale Park was pushed back. The tables, organized as one long table, marched down the centre of the room. Larry sat at the head, just beneath the hatchway into the kitchen.

Everyone was there: Faye, his son and daughter and their partners, his grandchildren, his sister, several close cousins, and some of his closest friends. He seemed full of good cheer, an effulgent host who enjoyed laughing almost as much as he enjoyed food.

He began, as always, with a short address, a meditation on Passover and its meaning. He never strayed far from his favourite themes: the eternal search for freedom, the need for vigilance to protect that freedom, and our responsibilities toward the oppressed and marginalized populations of our nation, like the First Nations and the Inuit. But he always had something different to share: some fresh nuggets of trivia about the Passover tradition he'd unearthed in his reading. He wasn't a religious man, but he was respectful of his people's traditions.

As he developed his theme, Judith, his daughter, snuck into the kitchen. Ostensibly she was there because the food needed attention. But that wasn't it. That's wasn't it at all. Earlier, her father had asked her two daughters, Jesse and Ella, to help him mix his infamously delicious chocolate cake. Which was most unlike Larry. He normally didn't allow anyone, even his beloved granddaughters, to interfere with his baking. There were benefits, to be sure. For him, of course, but more especially for them: a chance to lick the cake mix from the bowl, a chance to spend special time with Zaide.

He played it up as an adventure, this departure from the norm, an initiation into family ritual. But that was just his sleight of hand, his distraction, to draw the eyes away. He was simply too tired. He didn't have the strength to stand, didn't have the energy for the mixing. Judith noticed too that his appetite had disappeared. Normally there would be a lot of casual snacking before the meal itself, and Larry would have been one of the most ardent of the snackers. This year he'd hardly touched a scrap.

She could hear him, only a few feet away from where she sat, covering still. His familiar, easy laughter. His playfulness. And the poignancy of this pierced her heart almost more than the shock of seeing his weakness. She was overtaken by a presentiment she barely wanted to acknowledge.

Back in the lounge, as Larry looked out over the table at the assembled company, the action seemed to freeze. It was almost as if time had been frozen, as if Larry had been presented a gift: a golden frozen moment. And in this golden frozen moment a thought snuck into his consciousness. He couldn't say where it came from or why it came.

True, he was unusually tired and his appetite had been off lately. He hadn't been able to enjoy his food as much as usual. Most disturbingly, he seemed to have developed an intolerance of meat, which was unheard of. He was normally an unapologetic and enthusiastic carnivore.

But the tiredness, the nausea, the lack of appetite, it could have been anything. Nothing to worry about. Nevertheless, the thought, the same thought that was torturing Judith in the kitchen, refused to be silenced: *This will be your last Seder.*

CHAPTER 3

Bed

We don't speak of it, but the bedroom's surely the most intimate and vulnerable room in our homes. It's where we sleep, and when are we more vulnerable than in sleep? It's where we strip away the persona with which we clothe ourselves in our everyday lives.

When I suffered a heart attack in 2007 I didn't want anyone visiting me at my hospital bed, for these and other reasons. So when I showed up on the stroke of 9:30 of the morning of May 13, 2013, for my first meeting with Larry, I was surprised and a little nervous when Faye told me he was lying down in bed, and I could go into the bedroom and see him.

I'd known Larry for a little under six years, but I wouldn't say I knew him well. Natalie and I had been to the theatre with him and Faye, eaten lunch together, chatted at various Latner Centre events. We worked together on patient materials. I knew him well enough to write a brief character sketch in his profile on the Centre's website, but I wouldn't put myself in his inner circle.

I was relieved to find Larry was at least dressed. Perhaps it's my English background, this instinctive embarrassment over the pajama-clad. Larry had just had a new bed delivered; one of those fancy hospital-style beds with motor driven elevation for head and feet. On his bad days it was the most comfortable place in the apartment. There was a child's plastic drinking cup — the kind toddlers use, with a snug lid and a raised mouthpiece to drink from — at his side on the bedside table. This luminous interloper seemed utterly incongruous here amongst the dark woods and muted tones of Larry and Faye's bedroom. He picked it up between thumb and forefinger, his hand giant against the toddler-fist-sized handle.

"I'm reduced to this now. Drinking from a sippy cup. My hands are too shaky to handle a glass." He took a pull of water. The chemo dehydrated him.

He asked if I'd like a coffee. Faye brought it, but I was surprised it arrived solo. "You're not having one?"

"I can't drink coffee at the moment." It was another chemo side effect apparently. He could no longer bear the taste, though he used to love his coffee, was something of an aficionado. "Do you miss it?"

He shrugged, emitted a single chuckle. Almost apologetic, as if asking where to begin. Was it possible, was it wise, to document the things he missed?

I changed the subject. "Nice bed. New?"

"Yes. Our old bed wasn't going to be able to cope. Cost a fortune, but it's the most comfortable bed I think I've ever had."

It would be his death bed, I realized. An unbidden, uncomfortable, unwelcome thought. It almost seemed impossible, at odds with the mild spring sunshine bathing the suburban street outside Larry's bedroom window. The subject, I discovered, could not be changed. All subjects now led here.

The bed was the first accommodation to the cancer's despotic demands. Larry and Faye had yet to be visited by an occupational therapist, but the call to the Community Care Access Centre (CCAC) was one of the first he made after his diagnosis. In Ontario the CCAC arranges and co-ordinates health care in the home or in the community. If you want to be cared for in your home it has to be assessed by an occupational therapist, because you're probably going to have to make some changes: handrails in the shower, room to accommodate a walker, and possibly a wheelchair, and an increasing array of equipment. Your house or apartment may gradually mutate into something resembling a hospital more than a home, clinical equipment sitting side by side with your home comforts.

It had been a week and a half since I had last seen him at the party celebrating his retirement from the Latner Centre, and at least he was no longer the colour of a Stabilo Boss marker. But the chemo had clearly drained him of energy. His normally well-tended moustache was just the faintest bit less well tended, and his voice was thin and weak. It was usually driven through him by his infectious energy and enthusiasm. Today it seemed it was being forced out by sheer effort of will.

Larry had already started his chemo journey. I was surprised when Natalie told me he'd agreed to treatment. To me, chemo is an aggressive treatment whose aim is to cure. And it seemed clear it was too late for a cure. The cancer in Larry's pancreas was advanced and had spread to his liver. He knew, better than I, what that meant. So I was confused when I learnt he had still agreed to take a course of chemo.

Larry's oncologist, Malcolm Moore, was the director of the McCain Centre for Pancreatic Cancer at Princess Margaret Hospital. He's one of Canada's leading experts on pancreatic cancer. It would be difficult to imagine a better clinician for Larry. Larry admitted he wasn't sure if he was going to take the chemo initially, but Dr. Moore persuaded him.

"I was very clear with Malcolm and he was very clear with me. The reason for doing the chemo is to relieve my symptoms, help my jaundice, reduce my liver metastases, reduce any pain, that kind of thing. If I can prolong my life it will only be by a month or two anyways."

But at this point Larry wasn't sure if he was going to subject himself to any more chemo. "I'm so frigging sensitive to it," he said. He was on low dosages, and the drugs were mild, for chemo meds. "Nobody expected these side effects, including the neurological side effects. That would be unusual with the kind of little-old-lady drugs I'm taking."

It wasn't just the chemo fog. There was the weakness and the nausea too. He didn't want to eat or drink because he was nauseous most of the time. He held his hand out, turned it over to show me his palm. "See how pale I am? That means my hemoglobin's down by fifty percent. So I've replaced one problem, pale yellow, with pale. Just pale, not even pink."

Still, he wasn't definitive about giving up the chemo. "We'll talk about it. I can't do it at the same dose. I can't stand it. I would take it if it was a reduced dose, but will that reduce the efficacy? So am I just taking up space? Rather than doing anything. And they probably wouldn't know. They would probably want to do another three treatments and do a repeat CT scan."

We'd chatted for an hour, but his voice began to trail off. Not just quieter, but lacking Larry's usual attack. It was time to bring our session to an end, but before we did there was something I needed to say. I'd decided, before

I got there (but I was feeling the need to mention it even more keenly at that point), to issue some sort of apology. I'm not entirely sure what for: I'm English, we don't need much of an excuse. Less than two months ago Larry had been helping me with a story to raise the profile of palliative care in Canada. A cause Larry spent almost his entire career promoting. Now he was the story. It wasn't my fault, and yet I felt as if I'd carried out some kind of bait-and-switch on him.

And the words I came prepared to say seemed, strangely, simultaneously both more necessary and more stupidly insensitive. Still I bungled on, fully aware how gauche what I was saying sounded, but feeling the need to say it anyway.

"So," blundering right in, "this wasn't what I had in mind when we met at the Delta Chelsea."

Larry tucked his chin in, pulling his head back in a "did he just say that" gesture of incredulity. "It wasn't exactly what I had in mind either."

I tried to explain how these sessions might work. I'd hang out. We'd talk, probably for no more than an hour. If he was up to it we'd meet fairly frequently. At least once, preferably twice a week. At this point, of course, I was still thinking of this project as simply an article: something to illuminate the importance of palliative care for dying patients.

I had some ideas on where I wanted the story to go, but I didn't want to shape it too much. I knew I wanted us to discuss Larry's experiences of the health-care system, from the patient's perspective. I knew Larry would provide a unique point of view on the challenges he faced. My job, as I saw it, was to get out of the way, to try to paint the picture for readers. I wasn't sure what the story might be. That's the nature of this kind of story. It's no good trying to force your idea of the story upon events. Much better to allow them to speak for themselves. The story, in the end, would tell us what the story wanted. Which sounds a little mystical, but it's more pragmatic than it sounds. Neither of us knew what would happen, how events would pan out, what those events would show us. So I probably wouldn't know what the story was until the end. Maybe not even then. Maybe not until I started to write it.

It was another awkward moment. What I meant was we wouldn't know the true shape of the story until the story was finished, which in this case would be when Larry died. Even if I didn't mention death, he was standing at my shoulder the whole time. In the weeks that followed I got more used to his presence. Was able, from time to time, to call him by name and openly discuss him. This I attribute not to my courage, openness, and honesty, but to Larry's. Larry had spent a lifetime teaching others that the best way to deal with this particular unwelcome guest is to acknowledge him, invite him into the circle, and address him openly. Share the doubts, the fears, the tears.

It sounds easier than it is. There's an art to it. It's not something a novice will pick up easily. It takes work, and practice. Larry had thirty-five years of practice, and in the end he got pretty good at it, but even he caught himself falling into the same traps he'd seen his patients fall into. Even he had to catch himself.

He knew that total openness and total honesty could also be destructive. We must remember, he taught me, to protect our families and loved ones from the things they can be protected from, but equally, we must allow ourselves to surrender to them the things that they need in order to protect and help us.

I'm still a novice, and what I know of this I know because Larry taught me. But I hope we captured enough of it here to help others. Because, now that the story *has* ended, it seems much clearer what the story was and is.

It's the story Larry had been telling his patients for thirty-five years. The story he ended up living himself, through his own cancer death. The story of how to undertake this journey and see it through to its end with courage, openness, and honesty.

After I left Larry's condo building that day I walked part of the way home. I crossed St. Clair Avenue West at Bathurst and took the gentle ramp down into the Nordheimer Ravine. I needed to spend some time alone to think through the things we'd discussed. The popular psychology explanation would be that I needed to "process" our meeting. Perhaps that's the way it feels to some people, as if it were a meal to be digested, or a piece of code to be run through my core processors. That's not how it felt to me. I wasn't expecting a punch card to pop out of my head with an answer on it after wandering around Toronto for an hour. I wasn't looking for answers,

I was looking for equilibrium. That, and I needed to walk to work the tension out of my muscles. It seemed to pool there, somewhere between my shoulder blades. Walking loosened it.

I knew why. It didn't take a genius. Less than three years had passed since my eldest brother's death.

Larry and John were the same age, give or take a few months. And like Larry, John had been told his cancer was terminal when he was diagnosed and given a few months to live. There were other similarities too, if I thought about it. Both were, in their own ways, iconoclasts. Happy to strike out on their own path, if the path the herd was following didn't make sense to them.

Though Larry's situation was very different from John's. Our first meeting only served to highlight the contrasts. Larry was palpably ill. You could see it in the waxy pallor of his skin, and a certain dullness in his eyes, hear it in his voice. But he was still Larry. And he was relatively comfortable, sick as he was, in his own home, surrounded by the art he loved, looked after by Faye and Bella, the personal support worker (PSW) they'd hired to help.

I couldn't imagine a bigger contrast between the meeting I'd just had and the first time I saw John after he got sick. The utter devastation of it.

CHAPTER 4

Diagnosis

Beat upon beat.

Beat upon beat, beat upon beat, our lives inch forward, the increments of change so small we don't notice them. For months, years, we can maintain the illusion of our immutability. For illusion it is. Underneath, in the dark hidden recesses of our bodies, change is constant. Cell death, cell replacement: an unrelenting cycle of growth and renewal, of decay and decline. Until, at last, this quiet change that has been wreaking its havoc in the darkness announces itself to us. It may be quietly done. A persistent cough; nothing to worry about. Or, in Larry's case, simply a noticeable loss of appetite.

"You should have known."

Larry got used to it, in his final few months. He called it the Retrospectoscope. He said a lot of people used their Retrospectoscopes when he was first diagnosed. Forty-plus years a physician. Thirty-five in palliative care, caring for terminal patients who are mostly, these days, dying of cancer.

"You should have known."

It was everyone's first thought when they heard Larry was dying, that he only had months to live. The truth is, there were no signs. Not for the longest time. Pancreatic cancer is like that; asymptomatic. It's a stealth cancer, invading silently, leaving no discernible traces. That's why it's so lethal.

It's not a particularly common cancer. Your lifetime risk of getting pancreatic cancer is, statistically, about 1.5 percent. It's almost always the primary tumour, and it hardly ever metastasizes, but it has the worst survival rate of any cancer. The likelihood it will kill you if you get it is 98 percent. Which is why, although it's not very common (around 2 percent of cancer cases — there are 3,500 new cases a year in Canada according to Malcolm Moore), it's the fourth-biggest cause of cancer death in Canada.

Larry, who was sixty-six when he was diagnosed, was in the cancer's favourite target demography: 70 percent of all victims are over sixty-five. According to Malcolm Moore, we still don't know what causes it.

"You should have known."

And yet he didn't.

"I really can't track anything back before the new year. That's the strange thing. I wasn't losing weight. I didn't have any gastrointestinal [GI] symptoms. I didn't feel there was anything wrong," Larry said.

We were sitting in Larry's living room, the window to his back, the coffee table between us. It was our second meeting, and I'd asked him to recap for me the details of his diagnosis, but his answer didn't really satisfy me.

I pushed back. Surely there was some indication, be it ever so subtle? Was he certain he wasn't avoiding the truth? Maybe it rose to the surface of his mind every once in a while, only to be pushed away again? We've all done it, are all familiar with avoidance and denial.

But no, he said. No. It wasn't like that. There were simply no signs. "Sure, I was under a bit of stress. I'd just started a new job. So you're trying to figure your way through that, but the job turned out to be easy. It was a wonderful fit."

The new year, 2013, promised so much: the new job (even at sixty-six years old Larry was hungry for new challenges) and in February a two-week cruise to the Eastern and Southern Caribbean with Faye, sailing on February 7. It set off from Miami, sailing to Tortola in the British Virgin Islands, Barbados, St. Lucia, and St. Barts. "Just before we sailed we went down to Florida to see some friends of ours, and I started feeling full up easily. I didn't eat as much as usual. I didn't lose any weight, but I just found that while before I could sit down and have a honking big steak, now it was that size" — Larry's thumbs and forefingers met to enclose a modest oval — "and I felt full. My daughter-in-law was pleased because she's a vegetarian."

He didn't notice this intolerance to meat on the cruise. He ate well, gained two or three pounds. "We had a great time. It was wonderful. We met some nice people. We rested a lot. It was a small ship, had great restaurants, and we had a lot of fun. We really had a good time and when we came back I was feeling reasonably well."

But then he started to feel something was wrong. "You know, you get that sense of your body. I've noticed it before when I've had other illnesses … something's coming on, head for cover. And I felt, well, we'll see what happens."

It was then the food intolerance became much more severe. "I felt gassy all the time, and I started to have these funny abdominal pains I couldn't pin on anything. And some back pain."

Larry had suffered with back pain for years, arthritic pain, but this was different. It was higher, a low-thoracic/high-lumbar pain. His arthritis pain was at the bottom of his spine. And it was fleeting. It wasn't persistent. Not like his arthritis pain at all. "Then I lost weight like crazy, like a pound a day. And, after about two weeks, I started to get quite nauseated. I really only spent one day vomiting, which was interesting. But I just felt miserable. I felt tired. I did not feel right. To the point where I saw my family doc and we started the investigations."

His family doctor's initial idea was that, because Larry had some lower abdominal pain, he might have a bladder stone, "so we looked at that initially with an ultrasound."

The ultrasound found no evidence of bladder stones, and by the time the result came through his family doctor was on vacation, so Larry went to see an old colleague. Dr. David Tannenbaum is physician-in-chief of Family Medicine at Mount Sinai Hospital, and was Larry's boss when Larry was director of the Latner Centre.

"He took over. He said, 'We'd better get you investigated quickly.' When you're a doctor, you can pull strings a little bit. I was really sick. David thought I was dehydrated. So I went to see Hillary Steinhart [head of the Combined Division of Gastroenterology for Mount Sinai Hospital and the University Health Network]. This was on a Thursday morning. Hillary said don't have anything to eat or drink, we'll scope you today. So he did a gastroscopy the same day and then booked me for a colonoscopy the following Monday, and a CT scan the following Friday."

The gastroscopy and colonoscopy both came back negative. "They didn't find anything upper wise, didn't find anything lower wise, but you know, having gone through the colonoscopy, I was hating him with a passion. But I sort of knew by that time." One of the test results showed Larry's amylase was up. "Amylase is one of the pancreatic enzymes and it normally won't go up unless you have pancreatitis or something like that. But I was still nauseated, was not eating well, and driving my family crazy. Especially Faye. The big eater had stopped eating."

That same week Larry had another appointment at Toronto Western Hospital for another problem. "I've always had this tremor" — Larry held out his hand, and the tremor was quite discernible — "but it was getting worse. I'd noticed some things that made me think I had early Parkinson's."

He'd been waiting for an appointment in the movement disorders clinic for a while. It was just coincidence that it fell into the middle of his week of internal investigations. He saw Dr. Janis Miyasaki that Wednesday and she confirmed his diagnosis. "So it was like bang, bang, bang, you know, let's knock him into the ground."

But in some ways the diagnosis offered a ray of hope. Sometimes, Parkinson's causes a condition known as dysautonomia, "which just means the gut doesn't work properly." Larry seized on this: "We thought, phew, it's only Parkinson's. However, by the time I got the CT scan I really knew that Parkinson's doesn't give you these abdominal pains. I'd already figured out in my own mind this was radiating pain, because, of course, I'm the pain doctor." For years, Larry ran a weekly clinic at the Wasser Pain Management Centre at Mount Sinai Hospital.

The sense that something was wrong, something fundamental interfering with the smooth running of his body, haunted Larry for, he thinks, three weeks before his diagnosis. "You feel it in your body," he said. "I've heard that expressed by patients too, that when you're facing something mortal and severe, you know something's wrong with your body. I knew my body wasn't that nice working machine that it used to be. I may have been fat and out of shape, but you have a sense of the rhythm of your body and all of a sudden that rhythm is thrown off."

It wasn't something he could explain with his medical knowledge, although his first instinct was to try. He mused on the chemicals the body produces when tumours are growing, theorized that the body may sense this chemical shift, which feeds this sense of impending disaster.

Was he sure it wasn't just the Retrospectoscope? He leaned back in his armchair to consider the question, picked up his sippy cup, and drank. "I don't think so. I think I got a sense that my body was really in trouble for those two or three weeks, although it wasn't something that I could explain. I felt like my body was out of control."

Perhaps that's why people sometimes delay, rather than seek help. "They're afraid that something's wrong. Or they know that something's wrong and they're afraid to get the diagnosis. I heard that recently from a colleague of mine. Her partner knew something was wrong and just didn't want to upset her. This was a tremendous couple, and she knew something was going on in her abdomen. It turned out she had ovarian cancer and it was quite extensive. But she knew a couple of months before there was something wrong with her body."

It's bafflingly illogical of course, this fear of diagnosis. Your prognosis won't improve because you leave the problem undiagnosed. It's not the diagnosis that kills you, it's the disease. The faster you seek help, the better.* And yet we behave as if it's not there if we don't know about it. If you have something mortal, failure to seek help will not only make a cure that much less likely, it may kill you.

On Monday, April 8, a day that was etched in Larry's memory, Hillary Steinhart called first thing in the morning. It was a very brief conversation. Dr. Steinhart said: "I think you'd better come in and talk to me. I'm in the gastroscopy suite all day, but I'll take some time off and talk to you."

"I knew right away. The hidden message was there: I've got some bad news for you and I don't want to deliver it over the phone."

---

* It's not always the case that early diagnosis helps. There are certain conditions, and certain cancers, where an early diagnosis will have little or no impact on the outcome, and may indeed lead to more aggressive interventions, having a negative impact on the quality of life of the patient.

He got to Dr. Steinhart's office around 2:30 p.m. Dr. Steinhart left the gastroscopy suite and ushered Larry into his office and offered him a seat. Dr. Steinhart didn't sit behind his huge desk, he sat beside Larry, and he wasted no time in delivering the bad news. "He did a really good job of telling me in about fifteen seconds what I already knew, that I had pancreatic cancer."

Larry had been on the safe side of this conversation hundreds of times before. It didn't inoculate him from the impact of the news. Time, that elastic, malleable but ultimately stable measurer of our days, broke open, ceased to obey its customary rules. It was as if it were still running along, outside of him; as if everyone else was still pounding down its path, but whatever mechanism had attached him to that same treadmill had broken, disconnecting him. And into that silence, that sudden darkness, that crack that opened up in his world, poured all his grief and fear. The chaos of unknowing. As Larry described it, it felt like an implosion of all certainties. Followed by an explosion of fragmentary and jumbled thought: "Can this be true? Am I dreaming this? I don't know what to do. I must be in shock. I am in shock. What's going to happen — to my family? My job?"

Larry knew this is how patients respond to the news they have cancer. But there's a difference between knowing and feeling something bone deep. He'd delivered the bad news himself, had trained others on how it should be done. And his advice would have been no different, after he'd experienced it himself. There is no other way to do it than quickly, simply, and without ambiguity. There's also no way of delivering the news that will help the patient remember what you say afterward. "Once you hear you have cancer, the physician can keep talking for the next hour and the patient ain't gonna hear anything."

It was the extent of the disease that shocked Larry most. "I think it shocked Hillary too, because he tried to sugar-coat it a little bit. I asked him for a copy of the report and he became kind of nonplussed about that. Not because he wanted to hide it, because he knew. When I saw the report I was just decimated.

"I mean, I'd love to say I approached it the same way Timothy Leary, the LSD guru, approached it: 'Hey, this is wonderful. I've never died before.' But I think most people, certainly myself, just feel totally decimated. It's a reality I knew I was going to face at some point. It's just when it's right in your face" — Larry held his flattened palm an inch or two from his face — "it's very different. So there was the whole gamut of things from anger, to fear, to sadness, to tears. There were lots of tears. I mean, I'm not a guy who's used to doing lots of tears, but the tears were there. Faye wanted to come with me to the appointment and I'm glad she didn't because we both would have collapsed in tears in the waiting room."

Whether because intense stress makes us take refuge in routine, or because the news had numbed his critical faculties, Larry walked the two blocks from his specialist's office in Mount Sinai Hospital to his office in the Joint Centre for Bioethics on College Street. He was still clutching the report in his hand as he walked. He looked at it twice, but it still didn't feel real. He didn't stay at the office, just picked up his briefcase and took the subway home. "My daughter says I'm useless, I should have taken a cab. But I took the subway home because to me it's a sort of mindless journey."

Faye wasn't home. He knew she wouldn't be. It was barely 3:00 p.m. He wasn't expecting her for at least half an hour. He paced back and forth; an agony of waiting, knowing what he had to tell her, needed to tell her, yet not knowing how to. "I just tried to think how I was going to … because Faye was coming home afterwards … what I was going to tell her?"

Finally, he heard her key in the door, started toward it, to meet her as she entered. "I'm dying," he said.

"That will live in my mind for however long I live. The reality of just saying that, knowing what I knew, and watching my wife dissolve in tears, and then dissolving in tears myself. It was a measure of our relationship, but also a recognition of the pain we were about to go through. It was just a gushing forth of emotions: fear and love and anger and the surreality of things. That persists for quite a number of days afterward. It doesn't seem real."

I asked Larry if his knowledge and experience as a palliative-care doctor helped him better cope with his diagnosis. His answer was a little surprising, implying as it does that almost anyone can equip themselves under the same circumstances. Because he said the chief benefit conferred by his years in palliative care was "just knowing what to expect."

"As far as my emotions, that didn't come as a surprise: the depth of it was not surprising, the breadth of emotions I experienced was not surprising. The main thing my experience as a palliative-care physician taught me was that I did not want to see a prolonged period of two to three weeks of gnashing of teeth with my family."

The first thing he did was call Judith and David, his daughter and son. He was as blunt to them as he had been to Faye. "I'm dying," he said, as they answered the phone.

That same evening the entire family was summoned to Larry's condo "to make sure everybody understood what was going on." The good news was David was back in Toronto after living in Halifax. "Can you imagine trying to deal with this over the telephone or on Skype?"

That first instinct, what Larry called "the gathering of the clan," is something his years of experience as a palliative-care physician had taught him was absolutely vital. Too often the very opposite happens. The person who's sick withholds the information from their loved ones and families, to shield, to protect them.

"My experience told me I needed to help my family as well as myself," Larry said. It had always been Larry's philosophy: you don't just treat the person who's dying, you must treat the entire family. They're all grieving, confused, frightened. "So I really needed to make sure my family knew what was happening. I spent the first twenty-four hours just talking to important people in the family, people like my mother-in-law. We had to do it in person. We couldn't tell her over the phone."

He also knew he didn't need to panic and rush to get treatment the day after his diagnosis. "My experience as a palliative-care professional said just take it easy. It's not like there's a dagger at your throat, you've got time."

Larry started to get his affairs in order. On his own admission he was not the most organized person, and though he and Faye had talked about a will they hadn't quite got around to finalizing it. "I knew I had to get my legal stuff organized. Our lawyer had a copy of the will ready for six months, but neither he nor I had done anything about it. So I knew I had to get those medical and legal things done, some done right away, like power of attorney, and some started, like looking at what disability insurances I had."

All the while the faint suspicion that this was simply a big mistake, a case of mistaken identity, persisted. With one half of his brain Larry approached the end of his life in a logical, planned, and ordered way, "all the time having that surreal feeling like somebody's going to elbow me and I'm going to wake up and it's not me. I kept thinking it was a nightmare and I'd look in the mirror in the morning and I was the nightmare. It's the way it is. Now I look at my fuzzy hair and the nightmare is me." His shoulders started their subtle little dance, and he chuckled, more to himself than to me.

Of course, he didn't put off his treatment indefinitely. He got a quick referral, "a good referral," to oncology, "to Malcolm Moore at Princess Margaret. And he's a superb clinician, I really have a lot of respect for him. He didn't mince any words. He really laid out what could and couldn't be done. The good news was he didn't send his fellow or resident in to see me, because they often will do that. But he came in and gave me the low-down. Partly because Dave Warr (who is the person I shared the pain clinic with) was really after him, saying, 'This is an important guy, you'd better look after him.' But I've known Malcolm for years so it wasn't an issue. And then, because I was getting jaundice, all hell broke loose."

CHAPTER 5

Food

The Chelsea bun is a peculiarly English confection. Like much English food, it has been disguised to make it look unappealing to foreigners, resembling a building material more than a sweet treat. Baked to a mahogany brown, its surface will sometimes be marred by the odd charcoaled remains of a raisin or shred of lemon peel that has escaped the interior of the bun during the rolling process. They look like the cremated remains of houseflies.

Traditionally Chelsea buns were topped with a sticky sugar glaze, but the bakers of Britain's High Streets have long cut corners and now simply dust them with sugar. It's probably the only cosmetic appeal they possess, although it gives the first bite a gritty feel, much like the sandy bite of my grandmother's sandwiches on Margate beach.

But once inside, the Chelsea bun is full of surprises. The long strip of pastry that has been rolled into a squarish block to disguise its tasty goodness has been sprinkled with raisins, lemon peel, spices (cinnamon or mixed spice), and butter. So the bun's centre is moist and fluffy. Tastier, in fact, than its more popular and attractive cousin, the cinnamon roll.

When my twin sister, Sally, first visited him in hospital in April 2010, John told her the one thing he wanted most in the world was to taste a Chelsea bun again. He wanted it in the same way a pregnant woman might want a lump of coal to chew on: ferociously, insistently.

The fact that he couldn't have one, thanks to the large tumour in his throat, made him want it all the more. When John was first admitted to hospital the tumour was so large he could barely breathe, let alone swallow solid food. So he was hooked up to a nasal drip. Which bypasses the sense of taste altogether. You may never have been deprived of the sense of taste. You notice its absence. John sucked on mints and hard candy sweets for the stimulation of flavour, but what he most wanted, what he missed the most, was the taste of a Chelsea bun, and a pint of beer.

These are the things we lose. Everyday things. Things we've experienced thousands of times without pausing to savour them. These are the things that become important when they're taken away from us.

Most of my siblings stayed in the south of England when they grew up and moved away from home. Left London behind and became orbiting moons, attached to various compass points on the edge of the M25 motorway that circles London. Most, but not all.

I grew up in a crumbling Victorian council house in North London. My elder brother John was a mythic figure. He left home, and London, at fifteen to join the Merchant Navy. Every time he returned from one of his trips he brought with him talismans and artifacts from far-flung lands I'd only encountered in the pages of books: battery-operated tin monkeys from Hong Kong, shark's teeth and elaborately carved scrimshaw from the Far East, finely worked leather bracelets and necklaces from India and Ceylon.

On those rare visits home he itched to escape the confines of our crowded council house (or later, flat), inventing pretexts for trips and excursions.

A family outing, he said. A day of adventure. He would have been in his late twenties. Sally and I were almost a decade younger. Our brother Stephen was smack in the middle — half a decade separated him from both John and us twins. So we all spent the day on the Thames at Henley, rented a boat. Sally packed ham sandwiches, bananas, apples, grapes. John bought beer. He steered the boat upriver, away from the town, and moored it on a quiet little eyot near the left bank. We picnicked, batted drowsy late-summer wasps away with the backs of our hands, and watched dragonflies hover over the river, the only sounds the thrum of the insects and the deep-throated thunk of the inboard motors of passing boats.

After we'd eaten, John stripped off his T-shirt and, clad in his faded cut-offs, shallow-dived from the prow. We watched his bubbles rise and trail across the river. He was halfway to the other bank before he came up for air. My mother claimed he'd been born with a vestigial gill, which sometimes wept a clear liquid. Nobody had ever taught him to swim, she said. As a three-year-old he'd just jumped in the local pool and taken off. Fish-boy, she called him.

When he reached the far bank he turned without pausing and swam back; an effortless crawl that barely disturbed the water. As he pulled himself back onto the deck, he grinned. "That's a couple of widths, don't ask me to swim the length."

After half a lifetime sailing around the world, John finally met a woman whose allure was stronger than the sea's. When they first met, Phyllis lived in a council house on the outskirts of Liverpool, but together John and Phyllis dreamed of bigger and better things.

This was Margaret Thatcher's Britain. In the seventies the term *capitalist* had been an insult, hurled by ardent students at rallies. By the late eighties it had been rehabilitated. Capitalism enjoyed a renaissance, and home ownership was the primary doctrine in Maggie's Church of the New Capitalists.

Chasing the dream of home ownership, John and Phyllis moved to Oldham, a dour pockmark on the western edge of the Pennines. It was a boomtown once, a hundred and fifty years ago. The biggest textile mills in the world operated out of Oldham. At its peak, Oldham's mills spun more cotton than Germany and France combined. But that was more than a hundred years ago. In the middle of the twentieth century the mills started their long, slow decline. The last closed in 1998.

In the early 1970s Oldham was swallowed up by Greater Manchester, but it has missed out on Manchester's regeneration and gentrification. It's one of the most depressed and depressing places in the city. Most people are trying to get out of Oldham. My eldest brother was the exception. He moved in.

Property in Oldham was cheap. But their move was poorly timed. It coincided with a punitive rise in interest rates that priced them out of the market. John, by this time, had found himself work as a night watchman at the *Daily Mirror*'s print works in North Oldham. They arranged a council housing exchange and moved anyway.

They had thirty years together. John was as happy as he'd ever been. He finally had the family he'd craved (he treated Phyllis's children as his own) and the relationship he'd been looking for. But Phyllis died from an internal hemorrhage after a minor surgery in December 2007. John was never quite the same.

He started to complain about a pain in his throat in June 2009. He mentioned it in his weekly phone calls to my mother, but did nothing about it. He refused to see his GP, a man with an unfortunate dictatorial streak, which defies logic. The prognosis would not get better the longer he left the problem untreated; it only made a cure that much less likely.

Nobody knows why John held out so long. Perhaps it was because the doctor had made him stop drinking the last time he had seen him. Since Phyllis's death, John's drinking had turned from recreational to abusive. The doctor told him to stop or die. Perhaps he suspected it was something grave, and didn't want to face the diagnosis.

My mother, a sensei in the art of passive aggression, finally blustered, cajoled, and guilted him into booking an appointment.

John was a lifelong smoker. At five years old I knew what my parents did not: he regularly smoked behind their backs. He hid his ciggies and matches when he got home from school, and retrieved them the next morning. He had various hiding places: under the unruly privet hedge at the front of the house, nestled in amongst the tire repair kit in the saddlebag on the back of his bike, or in one of the mildewed old boxes stacked in the garage. He would have been fourteen or fifteen at the time.

His elaborate subterfuges didn't prevent my parents discovering his smoking habit. The row that followed simply drove his smoking further underground. I don't remember him ever attempting to give his cigarettes up during any of his sixty-three years.

The appointment with his GP didn't last long. The doctor asked John if he was still smoking. John answered honestly. "Then I can't treat you," the doctor said. And he proceeded to deliver a short lecture on the impact, financial and human, of smoking on the National Health Service. John never suffered lectures well, especially from authority figures. He didn't argue, or try to plead his case. He didn't utter a word. He simply stood and walked out of the surgery.* He hadn't wanted to go in the first place. The GP's lecture just gave him the excuse he needed.

---

*In the U.K., the offices of family doctors (general practitioners, or GPs) are still generally known as surgeries. The term is an anachronism, a hangover from a time long past, when GPs undertook simple surgical procedures. Obviously, GPs in the U.K. no longer operate on their patients.

The pain got steadily worse. His appetite, which had been poor since the pain started, all but disappeared. He abandoned meals more often than not, because it was too painful to swallow his food. He lost weight at an alarming rate. More disturbingly, there was now a discernible lump in his neck. But, worst of all, he was having trouble breathing. Finally, nine months after the pain started, my mother again persuaded him to seek help. If he wouldn't go back to his GP, she said, he should go to the Accident and Emergency department of the nearest hospital.

He was admitted immediately. He weighed just over one hundred pounds.

Those of us who live the span of an ocean away from our families know the terror of the unexpected phone call from home. Especially one out of normal hours: late at night or early in the morning. Mayhem lurks in that transatlantic static. You immediately imagine death or life-threatening disaster. In 2010 my mother was eighty-eight years old. If my twin sister, Sally, ever called from the U.K. a little later than normal, or even when I wasn't expecting a call, that hollowness would open up inside as I lifted the handset.

But there was nothing alarming about the timing of this call. It was a Saturday morning. Natalie was home, and I was probably watching the English Premier League. There are few Saturdays during the season that I don't. A good time to catch me, which must have been Sally's reasoning.

I don't remember much about the conversation. I didn't take notes, didn't expect to have to report it back. I know Sally wore her business voice, a more clipped delivery in a lower register, with fewer peaks and troughs in tone, and that I tuned in to that quickly. And I know she got straight to the point. "It's John. He's got cancer."

After that I took in very little. As soon as I got off the phone, Natalie, who had intuited the bad news from my side of the conversation, wanted specifics. What variety of cancer did John have? What stage? "All they've been told is that he has 'throat cancer,'" I said. "I don't know if they've even staged it yet, they're waiting for test results."

We headed for the computer. Natalie was an old hand at this. Our leading contender, after half an hour on the Internet, was a form of tracheal cancer called squamous cell carcinoma. Just a guess, based on a correlation with smoking, and the fact that it's more common in men over sixty. John was sixty-three.

Tracheal cancer is rare. Only one cancer in a thousand is a tracheal cancer, but of those, nine in ten are squamous cell carcinomas. So it was a pretty solid bet that's what John had. The prognosis for squamous cell carcinoma didn't look too bad. It rarely metastasizes from the larynx, and the five-year survival rate was very high at 98 percent, as long as it is treated early. A small qualification, but always a critical one.

As so often happens in families during times of crisis, our women stepped in to advocate for John with the doctors, the hospital, his nursing team. Sally and my youngest sibling, Julie, were hardly what you would call local to John's hospital. Julie had a three-hour drive to Manchester, on a good day on the M6 motorway. Sally's journey was at least half an hour longer.

On March 25, 2010, John had his first case meeting with his oncologist, which both Sally and Julie attended. Sally's email to her absent brothers (me, Stephen, and my younger brother, Barrie) was characteristically understated. "It doesn't look great for John. He's had a tracheotomy and they are draining fluid from it every so often as he has a chest infection. He looks dreadful." The oncologist had nothing to report. According to Sally, he "didn't have all the info." It was never made clear to us what this missing information was, or why it was missing at this first case meeting.

Evidently, case meetings happened on a Thursday. Sally was told John would have to wait until the following week for some decisions and a plan. But she wasn't sanguine. She didn't think he was strong enough to survive an operation to remove the tumour, or to undergo chemo or radiotherapy.

The case meeting the following week (appropriately, April Fool's Day) resolved nothing. The oncologist told John he needed an MRI (which Sally was told a week previously), but it was Easter, and it wouldn't be happening any time soon.

He was being fed glucose and a nutritional fluid through the nasal drip, and had gained about a kilo since admission. The medical team was happy with the slow weight gain. Putting on weight too quickly isn't good for the body.

As far as we could gather from the fractional information we got, the plan was to help him gain weight and strength, and look at treatment options once he was a little stronger.

The following week's case meeting on April 8 was attended by most of the family: Sally, Stephen, Julie, and my mother. They met John by his bedside to collect him and walk him to the small consulting room at the end of the ward.

Sally remembers him shuffling down the ward with the rest of the family surrounding him like a protective shield. "If I hadn't realized by that point how ill he was, there was no hiding from it then. He was so fragile. I asked him afterward how on earth he managed to get around before going into hospital. It's amazing how the human spirit enables you to do the seemingly impossible."

John's prognosis had dramatically worsened. The hospital had tried to MRI his neck and head on two separate occasions, but his chronic cough made it impossible for him to keep still enough, so they gave up. The oncologist had decided the cancer was too far advanced to treat. It was too late. John had lost the weight he'd gained since admission, and wasn't fit enough for chemo or radiotherapy. The tumour was too large (which I took to mean had invaded too much of his trachea) to be removed. They would give him a larger trach tube to help him breathe a little easier, and to help drain the mucous from his throat. They would also give him a gastric feeding tube, because the nasal tube was a temporary measure. Once they'd done that, all they could do was make him comfortable, manage his symptoms, and wait.

Sally walked John back to his bed. The others, stunned by the news, continued to pump the doctor for more information. "I remember holding his hands, and seeing the utter devastation in his eyes," she said.

"I clearly remember saying to him, 'You weren't expecting that, were you?' He said no, he thought that it was something he would be able to get through and recover from. I said that although it was a terminal diagnosis, that didn't mean he was going to die tomorrow, but I think for John it may as well have."

When he was first admitted to hospital, John was determined to fight the cancer, beat it if he could. The news that it was inoperable didn't, at first, fully register with John. When it did he became morose, depressed. "He started to distance himself from us all," Sally said. A phenomenon that's all too common in the dying, who seem to feel as if they've come untethered from the world, feel themselves floating away, carried by other tides, other concerns than the ones that drive everyone else's lives.

John's obsessions also evolved. At first he had craved the taste of a Chelsea bun and a pint of English bitter. The tumour had deprived him of his sense of taste and these were the flavours he missed the most. Now he had to come to terms with the fact that the tumour had robbed him of much more than his sense of taste. He had a new, much more insistent need, a need bordering on obsession. If the doctors couldn't do anything for him, he wanted to go home.

CHAPTER 6

Procedures

Larry thought the health-care system was trying to kill him. There wasn't the usual glint in his eye as he told me this, so I knew he was only half joking. "I feel like a sitting duck. It's like I'm in one of those shooting galleries and every time I go by somebody takes a potshot at me. It's dangerous territory."

He reached for his sippy cup, took another mouthful of water. It was about a week after our last meeting and Larry and I sat in the living room of his St. Clair West condo. Faye and Bella bustled around in the kitchen — we could hear them through the service hatch — and I had just set up my recording equipment on the coffee table that stood between our chairs.

Even though it was only "little-old-lady" chemo, it had clearly hit Larry's system hard. His eyes had none of their usual brightness, and he was gradually losing his hair. But at least he was no longer bright yellow. The jaundice problem had been fixed, but not before it nearly killed him. Twice.

What he suspected seemed unlikely. He was a VIP after all, a *Very Important Patient*. Not that he'd pushed to the front of the line, but everyone understood he was an important guy. If they were trying to kill Larry Librach, what are they doing to the rest of us?

He described this episode as "a two-week period of my life which was absolute horror, that I don't think I'll ever recoup.

"You want to replay it in some way, but the Retrospectoscope isn't that clear."

The pancreas, the site of Larry's primary cancer, sits in the U of the duodenum against the back wall of the abdomen. But the cancer had broken out. The pancreas is attached to the common bile duct (and ultimately to the liver) through the pancreatic duct. The cancer had invaded the end of the bile duct and obstructed it. When the body can't drain bile we get a variety of jaundice called obstructive jaundice.

"All hell broke loose. My urine was turning very dark, because when you're jaundiced you don't have an outlet [for bilirubin — a by-product of the body's breakdown of hemoglobin, the protein in red blood cells] other than your skin or your blood or whatever. So I was peeing out wonderfully fluorescent orange urine. If you took a UV light to it, it would fluoresce a bit. My granddaughter thought that would be a good idea. So they referred me to Dr. Paul Kortan at St. Mike's."

Dr. Kortan is a gastroenterologist, and is probably Canada's leading expert in a minimally invasive surgical technique called endoscopic retrograde cholangiopancreatography (ERCP). ERCP is a fairly routine procedure. It involves threading an endoscope (a thin tube with a light and camera) through the mouth, down through the upper gastrointestinal (GI) tract, and ultimately through the pancreas and pancreatic duct into the common bile duct.

It's not normally a long procedure, especially not for a leading gastroenterologist such as Dr. Kortan. Larry had known Paul Kortan for years. The two met and Larry was scheduled for his ERCP on the following Tuesday morning.

Larry was given a local anaesthetic, a spray to the back of the throat, to suppress his gag reflex, and an anaesthetic to knock him out. He was laid on his side on an X-ray table while Dr. Kortan fed the tube through his mouth and down to the bile duct. "You find the ampulla there — the opening of the pancreatic duct at the duodenum — and you can supposedly just thread a plastic catheter or even a wire stent if you can get in there, but they couldn't get in because the opening was blocked with either a lymph node or some tumour and they just couldn't get beyond that."

The procedure was supposed to take half to three quarters of an hour, but Dr. Kortan couldn't get through the sphincter — the opening of the bile duct. He tried to expand the opening by cutting it, but was still unable to get in. "I remember because they didn't give me enough anaesthetic to last the whole time." Two hours in, Larry began to recover consciousness. He was still on the operating table. "It felt like they were ripping my insides out."

Dr. Kortan apologized afterward. "He said I should take Wednesday off. I remember Wednesday as being a really good day, except I was getting yellow as a duck's foot."

Larry was confident the next attempt, on Thursday, would succeed. It didn't seem possible there could be a second failure.

"By this time I'm an old hand. I know the drill. Except this time I made sure to tell them to give me enough anaesthetic."

Dr. Kortan gave Larry enough anaesthetic, but he still couldn't thread the tube.

"That's so unusual for him. Everybody was just absolutely shocked."

Larry's oncologist, Malcolm Moore, was called in. "Malcolm got me admitted to the palliative-care unit at Princess Margaret and they booked me for an external drain at [hospital name redacted]."

This is a more invasive procedure that uses ultrasound to find a large bile duct. The surgeon then goes in to the bile duct using a catheter — a plastic tube with a metal guide wire. The tube allows the bile to drain, and it also allows a stent to be placed at the site of the blockage in the bile duct. A stent is an expandable metal sleeve that pushes apart the walls of the opening in the duct to open it up.

The next day was Friday, the fourth day of Larry's ordeal. He was in Princess Margaret Hospital but the procedure was taking place in the interventional radiologist's operating room in _______ _________.

Few people realize that the hospitals in Toronto's "hospital alley" are linked by underground tunnels, originally cut to provide direct access to the city's subway system. Larry made the journey through the underground tunnel between Princess Margaret and ________ ________ on a gurney. It's not the most comfortable ride. The tunnel's floor is uneven, and although the orderlies know where the worst spots are, and try to steer clear of them, in places it's impossible to avoid a rough ride. There was the usual banter back and forth between Larry and the orderly who wheeled him over. Sometimes being an insider has its privileges. Larry was in a buoyant mood when they arrived at the operating theatre.

"And the interventional radiologist [let's refer to him as Dr. X], came and explained what they were going to do. Although I already knew what they were going to do. What they do is try and find a large bile duct using ultrasound. Usually by this time the bile ducts are expanded. And then they thread a tube in, place a stent that opens it up, and everything's hunky dory. Well there weren't no hunky dory in all this."

Larry paused for a moment. Not to savour the point he's making, but to reflect. "I went along with all this. I knew the risks of the procedure, I signed the consent form they gave me." Not that there was really any choice at that stage. His jaundice was rampant. And, as he pointed out, the patient is very often hardly in a state to be signing consent forms.

They gave Larry the usual cocktail of anaesthetics and knocked him out. "It was wonderful," he said, "except ... he also had trouble placing the stents."

Again, the procedure was supposed to be quick. But again Larry was on the operating table two and a half hours. And again, they didn't give him enough anaesthetic. "The last half hour I was in absolute agony because I didn't have any anaesthetic on board. Apparently they'd cut something and I was haemorrhaging inside."

Larry remembered very little about what followed but the pain. He described himself as "three quarters shot" at this point. He didn't think he processed all the information he was given. He does remember Dr. X visiting him in the little recovery room after the operation to tell him "we couldn't finish the job but we'll do it tomorrow."

"Finish the job. Yes. Well." Larry said.

Larry rode the underground tunnel back to his bed at Princess Margaret. And there was, at least, some good news: the catheter was draining "copious amounts" of bile into his bile bag. I doubt any man has ever been happier to see the disgusting green/brown sludge filling the plastic bile bag at his side. "I was draining enormous amounts of bile — hundreds of cc's every few hours — which was relieving the pressure on my liver."

It was now Saturday morning, and the fourth day out of five that Larry had been inside an operating theatre. The fourth day out of five that he had been anaesthetized. Anyone who has had an anaesthetic will know it takes a day or two for the fog to clear. Imagine the impact of several days of anaesthesia in succession.

Once again Larry rode the gurney down the underground tunnel between the two hospitals. By this time he was in no mood for half measures when it came to anaesthetic. He'd already woken twice during the previous procedures. He was emphatic that he didn't want to do so again.

"I said, listen, give me enough anaesthetic. Don't fool around. I don't care if I don't wake up for half a day, just give me enough anaesthetic.

"I'm not a chicken around pain, but when you're lying there helpless on the table and they're saying 'just one more minute,' every second feels like an hour."

This time, mercifully, Larry didn't wake up until the procedure was finished. "When I came out of it he told me 'we think the stent is in place now.'"

Larry paused. "We think."

But there were complications. There was a lot of bleeding. Dr. X said he thought there was a blood clot in the stent. In a stent in the biliary system that's inconvenient, but not disastrous. It may block the stent for a while, but the bile will eventually dissolve the blood clot and clear the stent. The doctor said the tube was well in place and should be draining bile.

Larry composed his face into a wonky, bleary-eyed expression. "I'm saying, ooohhh kkayyy."

He rode the underground tunnel one last time. After that things got a little bit muddled because of the brain fog caused by the cocktail of drugs Larry had been given.

"I started to have pain, more pain, and I noticed that the stuff draining into this bag, which was supposedly attached to a nice plastic tube, was draining pale-green mucous-looking stuff that had sludge in it. It didn't look like bile."

Larry raised his concern with John Bryson, his palliative-care doctor at the hospital. Dr. Bryson spoke to Dr. X. Larry wasn't entirely sure what Dr. X told Dr. Bryson, but he thought he just assured him that the tube was in the right place and that the mucous-looking fluid was probably just some bile back up.

That was on Saturday. By Sunday Larry was completely miserable. "I had this thing draining. I was in pain, I wasn't feeling well. I was nauseated all the time. I could barely get out of bed. I was in a private room. My kids were there. Faye was there the entire time, but the day just sort of went by as very foggy and hazy."

On Sunday afternoon Dr. X decided to cap the tube, which is standard procedure. The stent was in place. It would probably not be draining bile to the duodenum because of the blood clot, but the tube would allow the bile to drain.

"All they do," Larry said, "is put this lock on the end of it." Once the blood clot had cleared, the stent would allow bile to drain to the duodenum, as it normally would.

"And they just left me, as they should, and we just waited to see what would happen. Initially it wasn't too painful. But then I started to get some pain. And then I started to get more pain. And then I started to get this really, really intense pain."

They gave Larry a two-milligram subcutaneous dose of Dilaudid (an opiate). He'd already been on a small amount of Percocet and Oxycocet to manage his pain, but clearly some bigger guns were needed. "So they gave me two milligrams of the hydromorphone [Dilaudid], which is equivalent to about five milligrams of OxyContin, so it should have been fine."

The drug was given subcutaneously, which doubles its effect. Still, the pain mounted. "So they gave me four to six milligrams of the hydromorphone. And I settled. I didn't have any pain."

There was just one small problem: "I wasn't breathing. I didn't have any pain, but I wasn't breathing very well. I was on oxygen. I was really gaga. I was confused, really drowsy, not sure what was going on at all." The breathing problems, confusion, and drowsiness were all side effects of an excess of opioids.

At this point nobody was clear what was wrong, but one thing seemed obvious — capping the tube had made matters worse. They uncapped the tube and called the on-call interventional radiologist. He told them to irrigate the tube. So they put a syringe on it and irrigated it as directed.

"Which just about sent me through the ceiling. I was in agony, incredible agony. So they gave me some more Dilaudid. God bless the palliative-care people, but I wonder sometimes about their ability to manage pain."

Which seemed a harsh judgement, until I remembered Larry's history. Like many of his colleagues who pioneered the "new" discipline of palliative care, Larry had to battle the mythologies and prejudice that surround opioids when he started out. Even today, some nurses and physicians retain these outmoded attitudes to opioids. These mythologies are at the root of most of the pain experienced by cancer patients. Health-care professionals prefer their patients to suffer pain rather than risk addiction or overdose.

Over the course of thirty-five years working with patients, Larry was able to dispel these myths and prejudices. He distilled his hard-won knowledge in *The Pain Manual*. His work on the management of pain was recognized when he was made the W. Gifford-Jones Professor of Pain Control and Palliative Care at the University of Toronto. If any physician in Canada understood pain management it was Larry Librach.

The Dilaudid seemed to work. Larry wasn't in pain, but as the afternoon wore on his condition worsened alarmingly. He started to jerk. He seemed to be having trouble breathing. His son, David, who was sitting at his bedside, noticed that he was wheezing. "By that time — it was late afternoon — they had given me chicken soup. I remember eating it and then about half an hour later I coughed up a big wad of chicken that was in my airway. I wondered why I was starting to wheeze." His breathing worsened, he stopped taking breaths for twenty seconds at a time. He had to be reminded to breathe.

Respiratory depression is a much-feared but rarely seen side effect of opioids. By then there was no question about it: Larry was overdosed on opiates, no doubt exacerbated by all of the anaesthetic in his system. Larry remembers very little about that day, Sunday, other than the incredible pain and the vague and shadowy presence of his wife and children.

On Monday morning Dr. X visited Larry and told him the tube would have to be fixed. Larry asked him, "What's wrong with the tube? You didn't tell me there was anything wrong with the tube."

"The tube is kinked," Dr. X said. "We're going to take you down to the operating room, but Monday's not my day to work in the operating room so my colleague's going to do this for me."

This, at least, explained why Larry had been wracked with pain when they capped the tube. With the stent blocked by a blood clot and the tube kinked, the bile had nowhere to go. It found the path of least resistance — and started to leak into his peritoneum. "You don't need a huge amount of bile in the peritoneum to cause problems. A small amount of blood in the peritoneum will cause a huge amount of pain. It's one of your defences against foreign bodies and strange materials being in body cavities. And that's where it leaked, and it was obviously a bile leak because it was just the most intense pain I have ever suffered.

"So, I'm a doctor. I listen to what my doctors say. They took me down to the OR and I remember his colleague, she was very nice and explained what they were going to do: they were going to pull back on the tube because it was kinked, it was in a V shape. They hoped as they pulled it back it would straighten out and they'd be able to work with that."

Larry didn't entirely know what happened next. He tried to piece it together, but as far as he could tell, as the doctor was pulling the tube it broke off. "Or so I understand, because I still haven't got the right story.

"The good news was during all this I was totally asleep. I don't remember anything. I woke up in their little recovery room, and the person who did the procedure actually didn't come out to talk to me. It was Dr. X who saw me. I wasn't sure what was going on. I was four sheets to the wind. I'd had enough opioids and I was probably toxic from all sorts of drugs by that time. I do remember Dr. X said, 'Some good news, some bad news.' The good news was he felt the stent was in place and that it was clotted off, but that would resolve itself. And it turned out that was right.

"But he said we don't know what happened to the plastic tube or the guide wire. Because accompanying the tube would have been the guide wire, which is supposed to keep it in place and allow doctors to manipulate it more easily."

He never found out what happened to the plastic tube. "I suspect it came out. I could have passed a small bit of plastic tubing in my stools without ever knowing. I wasn't going to go searching for that."

Larry's doctors looked for the guide wire with the X-ray, but they couldn't find it, either inside him or anywhere in the operating room. "The note I was given said the tube migrated north. Now north to me is a direction. In the body north is up. Why's it going north? It should be going south and out. So to this day I have no explanation of what happened to it."

Larry was taken back to his bed in Princess Margaret to rest and recover. The intense pain had gone, but he was still groggy and toxic from the opiate overdose. He settled in for what he hoped would be a quiet night's sleep.

At midnight on Monday night Larry woke. He was disoriented. He had no idea where he was, or why he was in this single room.

As Larry told the story, he realized, as he came to, the room was full of people. Faye, Judith, and David were crowded together at the bottom of his bed. They were holding his hands, his feet, crying and telling him it's okay, that they knew he was dying, that he'd said his goodbyes to them, that they would be good.

"And I thought 'Who the hell are these people? What do they mean I'm dying? I'm not dying.' I'm looking around saying 'Who called you in? Nobody told me I'm dying.'"

In his befuddled state (and despite the fact that he had no memory of having done so) Larry believed he'd called his son David on his cellphone and told him he was dying and that he should get his mother and his sister to the hospital as soon as possible. He continued to believe this throughout his final few months, and reported his version of the story to me several times. The truth was slightly different.

David and Judith had stayed at the hospital, although they had sent Faye home to get some rest in the evening. They noticed that Larry's breathing had become shallow, and that there were some long pauses between breaths. "He was cold; various other symptoms led us to believe he'd turned for the worse. We sat with him together and separately, talking to him and telling him how much we loved him. We really thought he may be dying, but he never was with it enough to express his thoughts. We were concerned enough that we called my mother back to the hospital, and then decided to call David Kendal in the middle of the night to see him," Judith said.

David Kendal came down and said, "I don't know if I can look at your chart, but I'm going to."

"He was concerned, but he didn't believe my dad was heading into his last hours," Judith said. Larry slipped back into sleep. The nurses made up a bed for Larry's son David, and Faye and Judith went home.

It's a measure of how disoriented Larry was at this juncture that he created his own story to explain the sudden arrival of his wife, children, and palliative-care physician in his room that night. That story was evidently firmly embedded by the time he spoke to me, despite the fact that he had no memory to base it upon.

By the time Tuesday dawned, Larry was determined to get himself home. "I said, 'You're going to kill me here if I stay here any longer.' I always said I wanted to go home. I'd already arranged for my palliative care through the Latner Centre. So I said I can't stay here. I've never had a good relationship with hospitals at the best of times when I've been admitted. I think partly because I know the system and partly because I can see what's wrong and partly because I feel like a duck in a shooting gallery."

But Dr. X apparently had other plans for Larry. He wanted to perform a procedure to put in another tube, so Larry would have a relief valve. "Which would have been a reasonable thing to do. But I said, I don't want him touching me.

"I don't think I would ever say that about any other physician. John Bryson, the hospital's palliative-care physician, was there at the time, as was one of the nurses, and I said, 'I don't want him touching me.' So we made quick arrangements for me to go home."

But Dr. X was apparently on his way over to see Larry. It sounds like a French farce, but Larry and his accomplices took the hospital's service elevators and escaped Princess Margaret by the back entrance as Dr. X was walking in the front entrance. By the time he arrived at Larry's bed, his patient had flown.

"So I made it home. I could have kissed the floor when I walked in. Of course, if I'd been able to get back up again that would have been another thing. But I was still yellow as a duck's foot."

When he returned home he says he was still more "out of it than with it."

"If it wasn't for David Kendal I think I would have stayed that way. David was amazing. We both recognized that I was toxic from the opioids. We agreed that I would start cutting them back.

"David didn't quite agree with the way I did it though." On his second night at home Larry decided to cut out the long-acting dose of painkiller (OxyContin) altogether instead of reducing his dose to thirty milligrams.

"At two o'clock in the morning I was in agony, absolute agony. We called 911. The ambulance arrived, took me down to Toronto General Emergency, where they weren't very busy at all. They saw me fairly quickly, gave me some medication, sheepishly waving their finger at me."

Larry learned a really harsh lesson. Even doctors need drugs. David came in next morning and said, "Yes, I wanted you to cut it back, but not cut it out." He told Larry to keep his hands off his drugs. "Faye is now my pusher. "

It took at least a week and a half for the clot to clear, and for the bile to begin to drain properly. Larry knew this because they were monitoring his bilirubin levels and it was ten days or more before there was a significant drop.

For those ten days Larry's bilirubin levels were a constant topic of speculation and debate in the Librach household. Larry's bilirubin became a barometer of his health, and by extension the happiness and mental tranquility of his friends and family. This obsession with Larry's bilirubin extended even to the Librachs' former nanny, now a family friend, who was staying with them for a short period.

"She kept writing us notes, asking me 'How's your Billy Reuben?'"

Some might say Larry was lucky. Setting aside the obvious irony involved in describing anyone with a terminal illness as lucky, consider how Larry's scenario might have played out for another patient. Larry knew how to navigate the system and get himself discharged. He was not likely to be intimidated by his doctors into a passive compliance to a procedure he didn't want and didn't believe was strictly necessary. He had already arranged for his own palliative care, at home, with a physician he had trained himself, from the palliative-care centre he'd cofounded.

One of the first times I ever met Larry was at a meeting of the Latner Centre's advisory committee. He joked that one of his main goals, as director of the Centre, was to ensure "it will still be around when I need it." I got the impression this was a regular part of Larry's schtick. Like all good humour there's a germ of chilling truth to Larry's observation: it was funny because we all knew the provision of palliative care in Canada is patchy and inconsistent.

Few of us have founded our own palliative-care centres to look after us when we're dying. What if Larry had been an ordinary person: Joe Blow from Scarborough?

The truth is, things might have been very different. He might not have found it so easy to escape the clutches of Dr. X.

Would his palliative-care physician in the hospital have collaborated with him and discharged him? Of course, hospitals cannot detain patients — let alone perform procedures upon them — without their consent. So theoretically anyone in Larry's situation can simply ask to be discharged. But how many would have the self-assurance to do so?

And Larry had the safety net of a palliative-care physician attending him at home. In Toronto, where you live matters when it comes to palliative care. If you're "lucky" enough to be within the coverage area of the Latner Centre, for example (as Larry was), you'll be able to arrange for one of their physicians to visit you at home. If you live the other side of an arbitrary boundary (in Scarborough for example) you'll be out of luck. The Centre doesn't have the resources or the mandate to provide coverage across the entire Greater Toronto Area. Other organizations can and will provide home-based palliative care, but again, the coverage is based on limited resources and geographical restrictions.

And, compared with other Canadian towns and cities, Toronto is well equipped to provide palliative care. The fact is palliative care in Canada is a patchwork of ad hoc services that don't begin to cover existing needs, let alone the demands that will be put on the system by our aging population. By 2036 over 3.3 million Canadians (roughly 10 percent of the current population) will be eighty or over. That's double 2016's figure.

If you die in Canada today it's much more likely than not that palliative care won't be available for you. Between 70 and 84 percent of all Canadians die without receiving, or having access to, palliative or end-of-life-care services, according to the Canadian Hospice Palliative Care Association.

So it's true. Larry was one of the lucky few who happened to live in the catchment area of one of the best palliative-care centres in Canada. But it shouldn't be a matter of luck. It should be a matter of policy, a matter of political will, that all Canadians have access to high-quality palliative care.

Imagine a Canada (or any Western nation) where only 16 percent of its pregnant women had access to maternity services. Where birthing mothers were expected to simply put up with the pain, or were abandoned by the system altogether. How long would we, would they, tolerate it? Yet people are dying in Canada with inadequate pain management, and inappropriate or non-existent symptom control.

Why does it matter? What difference does it make, if you're dying anyway? Will you even care when you get to that point? Larry's "escape" from hospital and his recovery over the following few days demonstrate why specialized palliative-care training matters. Larry was cared for by David Kendal. Larry and David had worked together at the Latner Centre for over a decade, and had become friends as well as colleagues. Larry was adamant that the outcome of his stay in hospital and subsequent opioid toxicity might have been very different had it not been for David Kendal's care.

CHAPTER 7

Donkey Derby

One thing was clear from Sally's phone call: if I wanted to see John before he died we would need to get to England quickly. We booked the cheapest flights we could find and flew out of Toronto on April 23, 2010 (a Friday). This gave us a few days in London to get over our jet lag. The following Wednesday we took the five-hour drive north in Sally's car.

We stayed overnight in a bed and breakfast in the Peak District. I wanted Natalie to see this corner of England. She'd seen plenty of the pastoral beauty of the south, but this is a different England altogether: grim but possessing a rough-hewn beauty. It seemed to match my mood.

We stayed at an old farmhouse tucked into a rocky crag. After we settled in, we went for a walk to clear our heads after our journey. We climbed the hill behind the farmhouse and walked the paths for half an hour or more.

As we topped the last ridge, the grey steel-and-concrete tangle of Manchester lay before us. Its grimy red brick and industrial chimneys smeared over the middle and far distance, its tower blocks nibbling at the edge of the country at the foot of the hills. The sun was already setting, but there was no golden glow in the sky, nothing to soften the effect. It was overcast with a hint of rain in the air. It seemed to me the city at our feet was sucking the light out of the sky.

It had been almost twenty years since I had last seen John. It wasn't my fault, it wasn't his; it's what happens when you live on opposite sides of the ocean. You lose touch. Life finds ways of filling your days with more immediate demands: the insistent chirrup of the email inbox, the unending carousel of dry cleaning, the mowing of the tireless and incessant lawn. It turns out we're distracted from the important stuff by the detritus of our lives.

Sally warned me what to expect: as my twin, she knows me better than anyone. She drove the car up to the grim Victorian hospital and swung it into a visitor-parking spot. I cracked the door open. The chill air of a Mancunian spring swirled in. It had rained all night, was still raining. As if the boarded-up houses and the decaying tenements weren't bleak enough, the low, grey clouds had leeched the colour away into a perpetual twilight.

Natalie was beside me. I took her hand as the three of us climbed the rain-slick drive. One foot in front of another, that's all it was. Just steps. But my feet were weighed down by a rising dread.

The automatic doors sighed open. The cocktail of dying flowers and carbolic couldn't mask a faint, sweet rottenness. Sally led us down a long corridor. Nurses bustled purposefully past. She turned in to a ward. Outside, a teenager in a gold-and-black tracksuit slouched on a plastic chair, texting, while his mother, or perhaps his sister, rocked a child back and forth in a grimy stroller.

It was ten minutes until visiting time officially started. I was naive, believed strict visiting times to be an artifact of a world long lost to us, an attribute of a freshly minted postwar National Health System, like starched white nurse's aprons, and the strange white head coverings they wore when I was a kid. I was about to push through the doors when Sally stopped me. "Visiting time hasn't started yet."

"Surely they won't make us wait? Not when we've travelled all this way to see him." Seven hours on the plane, five on the motorway. Twenty years. Ten minutes.

She smiled. "No harm in asking."

We snagged one of the nurses as she passed. Pled our case. Poured it on pretty thick, if I'm honest. Her eyes shifted from ward to corridor, to me, back to the ward, barely settled, but she let me finish. She pointed to her watch. "It's only ten minutes. We'll let you all in in ten minutes."

Sally didn't say I told you so, and she hadn't voiced her skepticism, but the telepathy of the twin told me this was what she'd expected. "We'll see if they say anything about there being three of us," she said.

"Let them try." We waited, mostly in silence, until the same nurse strode up to the door, exactly ten minutes later, swung it back, and announced, "Come on then."

Through the double doors, past beds on either side. Clusters of damp visitors and the pajama-clad sick.

Sally walked with a grim but familiar determination. Most people avert their eyes when life is too much to take. Not her. The clack of her heels on the linoleum-tiled floor counted down our final steps.

Halfway down the ward, a gaggle of nurses, five or six of them, stood around a nursing station. It seemed like an intruder in this cavernous Victorian room — a half-wheel of pine and aluminum, its modern lines and light wood facings at odds with the dark wood, grey linoleum tiles, and dingy greens of the ward.

The curtain of the bed opposite this nursing station was drawn. We couldn't see the patient until we rounded it. There was no time to compose my face. Just the dark, hollow shock of it, all in a solid rush.

His head was hunched. He was almost completely bald. A sparse apron of lank, greasy hair was all that remained of his golden curls. Several days' growth clung to the sunken wreckage of his face, like wrack on a ruined hull. His once-white T-shirt and his boxers hung loose on his emaciated frame. His joints seemed disproportionately large on his wasted limbs. There was a dressing at his throat, with a clear plastic tube poking through it. It kept him alive. He hadn't eaten properly for months, had trouble breathing. The tracheotomy opened up the airway below the tumour, but it meant he could barely speak.

My brain could not process this impossible transformation. This wretched old man, more skeleton than living being, could not be my eldest brother.

We gathered at the bottom of his bed — Sally, Natalie, and I. A look of confusion misted his eyes. His glance darted from face to face. He recognized Sally, but the haunted look remained when he saw me. I'd last seen John at our father's funeral. Blond and tanned, he'd towered over me. Just as he always had.

Donkey Derby day. A festival of idiocy, where "jockeys" attempt to ride reluctant and headstrong donkeys around a racecourse, and the assembled crowds hope for the donkeys to unseat their jockeys, or wander off the course and into the bushes, preferably with their jockeys — trying to steer them back into the race — still aboard.

I remember the callouses on John's cigarette-stained hands. The modest iron gates of Alexandra Palace's racetrack had swung wide open to admit the crowds. The crush as we squeezed through the gates must have been enough to worry him, and he had reached for my hand, which was a little demeaning. I was too old to be holding hands in public. I must have been at least eight or nine by then, maybe even ten. But I took his hand anyway. And I remember the frisson that ran up my arm as it closed on mine, the shock. It was hard as leather, with nubs like studs on his palm, where the finger joints were. Hard as it was, and strong too, his grip was gentle.

He let my hand go once we were clear of the crush at the gates, and we wandered, side by side, toward the racetrack. The first girl stopped us yards from the gate.

"Hi, John."

"Sorry, do I know you?"

"Not as such. I'm a friend of Pat's."

He stopped, chatted for a minute or two, and moved on.

Seconds later we were stopped again. This time it was three girls, giggling in a huddle before one of them got up enough courage to wave and call, "John." He stopped and they approached.

"Who's your friend?" she asked. At eight I had no interest in lumpy, giggly girls and their obsessions. But I remember her vacant expression, her baby-doll eyes, lined in black, and her pouty pink mouth.

"My kid brother."

"He's going to be a looker when he grows up. Such pretty eyes."

Much as I wished it to, the ground did not open up to swallow me.

Our progress was glacial. We were stopped every few steps by a girl he knew, or the friend of a girl he knew. He took it all in stride. He was polite, chatted to them all, before drifting back toward the racetrack.

"What do they want?" I asked at last, frustrated at all the interruptions, and eager to get to the Donkey Derby itself.

"Search me, kid," he said.

The nurses had been teaching him how to use his fingers to block the tube in his throat a little, and force some of his exhaled breath over his vocal chords. He had to huff out words, each sentence a suffocated whisper that could barely be heard. Sally leant her ear closer to his lips. They were red and moist, an almost startlingly livid tear in his gaunt face. She angled her head toward us and smiled. "He said, 'Who's the bird?'"

Of course, he'd never met Natalie, my Canadian bride. He took my hand — still much smaller than his — and squeezed with a shocking strength. I introduced her. He smiled, and for an instant I saw that mischievous old sparkle quicken in his eye. He nodded, whispered, "Hello, love," and coughed — a phlegmy rattle, accompanied by a clammy sucking from the tube in his throat. A fat stream of mucus oozed from the tube and dribbled onto the white dressing. Sally was up and wiping it away before he'd even noticed. He was particular about his appearance once.

The nurses clustered around the nursing station gossiped loudly about a colleague, or a patient. Bursts of laughter punctuated the quiet of the ward. Patients and visitors tend to whisper to one another, as if raising their voices might break whatever spells were being cast here, but nurses didn't seem to respect such reverent superstition. One of the five peeled away and ambled across the ward toward us. She had the look of a traffic warden, relishing the prospect of the ticket she's about to issue: the rolling, wide-legged gait, the eyes that take in her audience as she passes, the watch-this-kids sneer. She said something to Sally, but I was at the head of the bed and didn't hear it. As she ambled off down the ward, I walked to the foot of the bed.

"What did she want?"

"She said there's only supposed to be two visitors per bed."

Fortunately I don't have superpowers, because I swear I would have punched a hole the size of a heart into the nurse's back if I'd had laser vision.

"Does she realize we've flown over from Canada to see him? She knows he's dying, right? That I'll probably never see him again?"

"Them's the rules." She reached out to me, put a hand on my arms, clenched tightly across my chest. "Don't worry. I'll deal with it."

She was managing me. Because an incendiary relative using his fear and frustration as a launch pad to invective would not have been the slightest help to John.

I've never forgotten that nurse.

I turned my attention back to the bed. "Taken the diet a bit far," I said.

He smiled. He wanted to speak again. His hands fluttered at his throat. I leant closer. The stench, dense and sharp, hit me like a punch. "I suppose I won't see you again, for a while," he whispered.

I squeezed his hand. He returned the pressure.

When I was a kid I watched him play chicken with his friends, a gang of riotous and ill-kempt glory seekers, in hand-me-downs and hand knits. They'd range their bikes along the pavement and wait. To John's left, snot-nosed Joe, cowlick flying proud. To his right, bug-eyed, buck-toothed Jeffrey James. He of the eternally scabrous knees. The side roads around our council estate were sparsely populated by cars in the late fifties. Sometimes they'd have to wait ten minutes or more for a passing motorist. The last to cross in front of the car without getting hit was the winner. John was always last to cross. I watched him once to work out how he did it. The other kids all watched the car, waited until they could wait no longer. John, pedal cocked, watched the pedals of the other kids' bikes. He didn't stomp down on that poised pedal until the last kid flinched and fled across the road.

"No," I said. "Not for a while."

CHAPTER 8

Callous

A callous develops when our skin is injured or (more likely) when it's stressed by constant friction. Guitar players develop callouses on their fingertips because of the constant pressure and movement of the string against their skin. It's one of the first requirements of the apprentice player, that they push through the pain of fingering the guitar strings until the comforting extra skin of the callous has grown. There's a sense of protection packed into the notion of the word, an insulation from pain and suffering when a body is subjected to the same stress over and over again. Were it not for the skin's ability to protect itself in this way it's likely the average guitarist would finish every gig with their fingertips shredded and bleeding.

This ancient, primary meaning of the word (*callosus* in Latin means hard skinned) was appropriated, sometime in the fifteenth century, and applied to insensitive or cruel behaviour. Initially it was a metaphor, but it's been used in this sense for so long now that it's easy to forget the word's origins.

The extension of the word to the psychological domain is understandable. Just as the skin thickens to protect itself, so the psyche develops an unfathomable ability, when continually confronted with scenes of pain and suffering, to protect itself by ceasing to see it, which allows it to cease to feel it too. What begins as self-protection may harden into cruelty and heartlessness. Because what the metaphor fails to capture is something fundamental to the human condition. The universal propensity to empathy, to feel the hurt of others, to sympathize with it, to wish to alleviate it because we understand the suffering involved. It requires a leap of imagination: the ability to put yourself inside the body of another human being. Psychological callousness involves a failure of the imagination. The sufferer can't (or won't) allow themselves this luxury of fellow-feeling.

This callous of the psyche allowed a nurse to try to turn me away from my dying brother's bedside because of hospital rules. It impacted Larry too, during his illness: indifferent, self-absorbed health-care workers who put the demands of the system over the needs of the patients within it.

There was a certain irony about the place Larry chose to tell me this story. We were in the Librachs' sitting room, in the armchairs in the television corner. The wall beside us was Larry's tribute wall, a patchwork of certificates, awards, and commendations from around the world, recognizing his work.

It was way past time for us to have our discussion on the defects and blemishes in Canada's health-care system, but it was a conversation I'd been avoiding. It's hard to say why. Perhaps because it's hard to put a human face on a string of statistics and complaints. Perhaps because the stories of drama and conflict that the data contains are too deeply buried to be easily found.

Typically, Larry's first thought on the system had nothing to do with the economics of it. "Where do you start?" he said. "First of all I sometimes wonder if we have a system, which to me is an integrated series of parts working together very efficiently, like an engine in a car. You have the rings here and the pistons there and they're all working together and if one starts to go awry the whole thing breaks down. Unfortunately [in the health-care system] we have a bunch of pieces that sort of link together, and although they may be interdependent, sometimes they act very independently. But overall the system is not person-centred. It's more centred on the disease, on illness. It's not centred on the person or their family. The system needs to have a sense of loyalty from the employees who work in it. I think a third of the people [in the health-care system] are just doing their job. They couldn't give a damn about whether they're processing chocolate mints or people."

I asked for an example to illustrate his point. He had one at his fingertips. "Like the woman at reception at Princess Margaret Hospital." Larry needed his hospital card. "She was sitting, filing her nails. I asked for the card and she castigated me: 'They should give it to you at chemo. You better go upstairs and get it there. I'm closed now.' They close at 3:30. I looked at the clock behind her. It was 3:27. I looked at my watch. 'It's 3:27,' I said. 'I need my card please.' 'Well,' she said." Larry's mouth pursed in imitation of her irritated moue. "She went on babbling," but she also processed his hospital card. "It took her maybe thirty seconds to produce the card." It took her less time to make the card than it took her to argue about making it.

It's trivial, but it demonstrates his point. The development of a psychological callous may be a defence mechanism, but it's a short-sighted one. One day Larry's reluctant receptionist may find herself in Larry's situation. And if and when she is, the quality palliative-care service that looks after her will be due in large part to the efforts of the man who was standing in front of her. The man for whom she couldn't spare thirty seconds.

"It's people like that. The person who was trying to take my blood from a tendon. I knew she was trying to take blood from a tendon, but she kept blaming me. 'You gotta straighten your arm more. You gotta do more.' And I said, 'I know my veins. I don't have a vein there.'

"In the chemo suites people are really good. There may be a maelstrom around you, but your personal nurse is really good … though it's hard to know each member of the team. But people need to approach their job like they're really trying to help people. Most people are in health care because they want to help people." Larry thought it wouldn't hurt if health care adopted some communications and motivational skills from the retail sector. "We were in Yorkdale yesterday, first thing, and the stores all gather their employees: 'This is what's on today, this is what we have to look for, these are the things you need to have, we've had complaints, this is what you need to do.' Instead the hospital staff fling the doors open and a horde of people go in for their clinic appointment. There has to be a sense of belonging and a sense of pride in what you do."

Larry cited a study by Cancer Care Ontario that showed 40 percent of oncology professionals feel demoralized. "There's a variety of reasons for that, but it will translate into poor patient care. It had to do with people feeling responsible when patients die of cancer. Well, people die of cancer because people die of cancer. They were going to die of cancer. Your role is to care for them, to comfort them, and to prolong their life if you can, to cure them if you can. But you can at least comfort them and look after their suffering. That has to do with education and orientation. Most oncology professionals don't get enough orientation. They're told this is what you do for infection control and this … and this … and this …" Larry chopped the job down into sections with his hand, breaking it down into tasks that need to be performed. "But there's not a sense of supporting people, there often isn't a sense of working as a team.

"In the GI clinic I get the sense there's a real team there. Malcolm Moore is at the pinnacle, but they work as a team. The nurses all know each of the patients. They all sit down and look at who's coming to the clinic [that day]. It makes a difference, treating people as people, welcoming them.

"And we're not mindful of people's time. When I was in family practice I had a patient who was CEO of a large corporation. He developed lung cancer. I sent him to see a respirologist. He sat in the waiting room for about two hours before he was seen by this physician. This was a guy who used to fly up to Pearson from his house in the Bahamas for his annual physical. Not a guy to be toyed with. He asked the physician, 'How much do you make for a consult?' He told him. So he sent him a bill for almost $90,000. He said, 'This is what the two hours you made me wait in your waiting room is worth for me.' Now he did it tongue in cheek, but we don't value people's time, not just CEOs."

Larry recognized there are sometimes problems scheduling appointments. For years he ran a pain clinic, and the scheduling was a perennial headache. "Arranging appointments at appropriate times was an issue, because we had people who needed to go to other clinics. There was one patient who had his first appointment at 9:00 a.m., another at 1:00 p.m., and then usually an appointment with us at 4:00 p.m." Often, Larry could see the patient early, but if he couldn't fit him in, the poor man, who travelled down from Sault Ste. Marie every week for his treatment, had to spend the whole day at the hospital. "And the guy could barely walk and breathe. It's what we do to people. We've closed the Princess Margaret Lodge now. People who were being treated used to be able to stay overnight. Not anymore. Budget. People have nowhere to stay. They take a hotel room or they sleep out in the car. Somebody was telling me the other day that a friend of hers came in for breast cancer treatment. She'd bring a sleeping bag and pillows and sleep in the car while she waited for her appointment, because there was no other place for her to sleep or to get comfort. There are no chairs in the atrium of PMH."

A little empathy, Larry thought, would go a long way. "We should remember that we could be in their spot. We should try to see the world as they see it, because it's very frightening. If you're semi-literate and you're coming from one of the northern areas, or you're Native Canadian or Métis, you're entering a culture you may not have any idea about. It's very frightening, especially if there's nobody there right away to help you. We just don't value people in that way. I took the job at the Canadian Partnership Against Cancer [CPAC] because of this issue of person-centred care, which involves the patient, the family, and the health-care providers.

"Our health-care administrators are so divorced from the bedside they don't see what's going on. They think they're producing GM cars. This spreadsheet approach drives me crazy. But on the other hand the government forces their hand. The government's discovered pay for performance. Well, what's performance? How do you measure it? How do you measure humane care? That's been one of the bugaboos about palliative care. How do you measure the value of somebody going to sit with somebody in their home to hold their hand, or to explain things, or to help them with their fears? There are no measures for it." The figures on how much you can save the health-care system by avoiding hospitalization are easily obtained, Larry pointed out, "but how do you measure humanity in that? We measure patient satisfaction, which if you're expecting nothing and you get nothing it's a hundred percent satisfaction. 'Hey, this is good, I got exactly what I expected from the system, which is nothing.'"

Even the architecture reflects the system's biases, Larry said. "Architects who build hospitals shouldn't be the prize-winning architects who build apartment and office buildings. You have to have a special sense of who people are and treat them properly. I'd like to take the architects of Princess Margaret Hospital and throttle them. Tell them to sit in that atrium. There are not enough chairs. There's a lot of noise. There are a lot of competing smells. The signage is poor. When people are waiting for blood tests they have to filter out into the hallway. You have to get up and lose your seat to find out what number is being called. As soon as you walk into a place it should be welcoming. Walk into Princess Margaret, the Murray Street entrance. It's dark. It overhangs the road. No sunshine gets in there. The lighting is terrible. It's hilly. You almost have to be in perfect health to push the swing doors open. On the University Avenue side there's no clear evidence of a wheelchair ramp, although there is one. Getting in and out of the place is awful. You're immediately met with food odours when you walk in either entrance. Tim Hortons on the University Avenue side and Druxy's at the Murray Street entrance. So if you're nauseated from your chemo and you're coming in for your second day of chemo it doesn't help to enter either side. The elevators are crowded. They don't hold enough people. The room where they take your blood is low ceilinged, low light. You don't want high-intensity lights, but you'd like some softened lighting. The chairs are uncomfortable and there are not enough of them.

"The number system works, I guess, because it keeps people in line, you have to do that, but it doesn't prioritize people who have to go to their clinic in an hour. It sometimes takes an hour and a half to get your blood taken. So if you're coming from Gravenhurst, you drive in in the morning, already you're going through Toronto traffic to get downtown for 8:00 a.m. because your appointment's at 10:00 a.m. You arrive to get your blood drawn at 8:00 a.m., but it may not get done until 10:00 a.m. Or your appointment could be at 3:00 p.m., so you have to spend the whole day. You shouldn't have to do that. You should have your blood taken right outside the clinic. There's no reason for blood to take as long as it does. We have autoanalyzers now.

"All these systems need to work for the benefit of the person, the family, and the oncology professional. They need the blood work as quickly as possible. I heard one of them the other day saying we don't get the blood quick enough. Well plain white count of hemoglobin, which is what most of them want, is a two-minute test that can be done anywhere.

"I haven't been on the wards of PMH, I've been on the palliative-care unit. It's well-designed and would be a reasonable facsimile of a ward. But if you look at Mount Sinai, which is redoing its wards, or Toronto General, we still have a lot to learn about movement of people in places like that. The system is not welcoming to you when you come through the door. It lacks effective information exchange.

"They give you a big information binder when you first come in, *My Journey*. You look in there, and first of all it's confusing and it's not in your home language, and according to one of my oncology colleagues most of the stuff in there is mythology anyway, so not very helpful. There should be a volunteer welcoming everybody coming into the centre, helping direct them. If it's your first visit you should at least be offered a tour before you come, to make things less frightening. There should be a place for you to sit down. I've been to American hospitals that are absolutely outstanding in the way they welcome people. You feel like you're in a hotel not a hospital. There are ways of doing it, and they're not any more expensive than what they spend already at Princess Margaret, which is a good hospital."

But the big issue everyone in health care is worried about has nothing to do with architecture or systems. It's all about demographics: the so-called Silver Tsunami of baby boomers that will soon overwhelm Canada's health-care system. Ontario's auditor general's 2014 report on palliative care provided a snapshot of what this Silver Tsunami is looking like as it gathers strength: "People aged eighty-five and over constituted the fastest-growing segment of Ontario's population between 2006 and 2011, with their number increasing by twenty-nine percent over that period. The number of people aged sixty-five and over is expected to more than double from two million in 2012, when baby boomers began to turn sixty-five, to over four million by 2036, when seniors will constitute twenty-four percent of the population."

Larry believed the threat of this wave of the aged is being overdone. "I think we're going to be overwhelmed by this idea of the Silver Tsunami, the idea that us older people are going to overwhelm the system. It's nuts. We know that we're going to have more elderly. But there's a commercial on TV by Heart and Stroke that says 'the average Canadian will spend their last ten years in sickness.' Well let's look at those figures. Ninety percent of us will die with two or more chronic illnesses, which will probably include high blood pressure, osteoarthritis, and some heart disease, diabetes, or something like that. But we may not be suffering. We may be very productive citizens. It's only in the last two years of life that the elderly really provide a challenge to the health-care system, and then most die off very quickly. But we tend to think of the nursing home people, who don't die off quickly. They're a particularly sad burden for us, because we don't know how to handle them except to warehouse them. But we're so caught up in the baby-boomer problem. Baby boomers like me, until I got my cancer, we're very productive. Sure I've got osteoarthritis and high blood pressure. I take my medication. I'm fine. We're so wrapped up in blaming the elderly. When you look at health-care costs, the reality is the greatest growth is in the thirty-five to fifty-five age group. They demand more care, more specialist care, more interventions, more testing, more, more, more. I think blaming the elderly is a really good thing, but what are you going to do with it?"

Clearly, Larry was being ironic. He didn't think blaming the elderly was a good thing at all, and when he asked what we were going to do his point was that the system's not simply going to euthanize the old for burdening it with expense. His point was we treat them like off-scourings. We see no value in them. "People who are sixty-five don't suddenly turn to mush. The system has to recognize the issues with the elderly, but not be overwhelmed by them."

Larry was also bothered by the way what he called "the cancer system" and the media manipulate public opinion by portraying images of cancer sufferers. "That comes from the whole breast cancer schlamozzle. It makes people very angry because it's not the reality. Most people who have breast cancer are elderly, not young women. In fact, a lot of the young women who are diagnosed with breast cancer are false positives. There's good evidence that we over-diagnose breast cancer in women, just as we over-diagnose prostate cancer in men. They have a little island of precancerous cells and we call it cancer and everybody goes crazy. But the vast majority of people who are dying of cancer are over sixty. The typical cancer patient you see profiled is a young person, a kid or a young woman with cancer, because it tugs at the heart strings. An eighty-five-year-old woman dying of lung cancer? Well, you know it's her time."

Why does it matter? If profiling helps raise money for research, can it be a bad thing? "Except we're in danger of ignoring the elderly. How do you help them cope with their cancer? Maybe we do too much. Maybe we offer too much. Maybe we offer them chemo that can kill them. Are we dealing with the quality of their life versus quantity? People are not given the choice of no treatment when they should be given the choice. You don't have to have treatment."

It's an excellent point. There's a growing body of evidence that suggests heroic measures to save the dying are crippling the health-care system. Most (72 percent) of the spending on end-of-life patients is for acute-care services, a figure that excludes stays in intensive care units. This is an Ontario statistic, but it's a similar story across Canada. Even south of the border, in the U.S., the overwhelming majority of end-of-life spending is focused on spending to save the dying at all costs.

In Ontario, over 70 percent of deaths occur in hospital or long-term care homes. According to the Canadian Hospice Palliative Care Association this is a little lower than the national average, which, as of 2000, was 75 percent.* Shockingly, almost half of all deaths in Ontario (46.1 percent) occur in acute-care settings, which works out to nearly 65 percent of all hospital deaths. One reason for this is our cultural bias for keeping even dying patients alive. It's not uncommon for dying patients to be admitted to acute care from the emergency department.

And yet the vast majority of Canadians say they want to die at home. Studies from around the world have shown that when terminally ill patients are being treated at home they're more satisfied with their care, more likely to die at home, less likely to visit the emergency department, and less likely to be admitted to hospital. Less likely, in short, to be a burden on the health-care system.

It's something that has perplexed me for years. You'd think the health ministries in every province would have embraced Canadians' desire to die at home, because it's far cheaper for the health-care system to care for them at home. It's also safer for the patient, Larry pointed out. Costs will vary by illness and across provinces, but according to Ontario's auditor general, in Ontario the cost of providing palliative care in the last month of a patient's life averages around $1,100 a day in an acute-care hospital bed; $630 to $770 a day in a palliative-care unit bed; $460 a day in a hospice bed; and under $100 a day at home.

---

* Canadian Hospice Palliative Care Association, "Cost Effectiveness of Palliative-Care: A Review of the Literature."

Larry said, "Our home-care system is broken. Broken, broken, broken. The system needs a good swift kick in the butt. But because it's not under the Canada Health Act the provincial government isn't forced to do anything about it.

"I haven't experienced the home-care system as much myself. I have a home-care nurse that comes in once a week, and I have some equipment, but I really haven't needed much help. There's not enough money in home care, as in most areas of health care, but that's the government's fault. They keep talking about pouring more money in, but there's no more money. The home-care budget is the same as it was twenty years ago, yet the number of patients has doubled or tripled."

It's hard to verify Larry's numbers. The Ontario's auditor general's own report in December 2014 pointed out: "The total amount of Ministry [of Health in Ontario] funding used to provide palliative-care services is not known." However, a report published in March 2015 confirmed that the number of people receiving home care has doubled since 2003–04.* Over this same period, funding for home care has only increased by an average of 5.6 percent annually. "The Ontario Association of Community Care Access Centres reports the number of long-stay, high-needs clients it has been serving has increased seventy-three percent since 2009."

"The resources available for home care, like personal support workers, have declined," Larry said. "The number of things that you can get, the length of time that you can get things for.... And the system rejected specialization, which would have been best for palliative care. We could have served many more patients. Every nurse has to be a generalist in home care. Some agencies still believe it's absolutely wrong. The government's trying out a number of different models now, but there's a gap between care in the hospital and care in the community.

"And the government keeps saying we are going to emphasize home care. What they mean is they are going to stop you from coming to the hospital, but it doesn't mean they'll put anything on the other side ... maybe they'll put armed guards around the battlements of hospitals ... and prevent you from getting inside."

---

* Government of Ontario, "Bringing Care Home: Report of the Expert Group on Home and Community Care."

The Canadian Hospice Palliative Care Association made a similar point in its 2010 policy brief on hospice palliative care: "Although there has been a conscious effort on the part of health systems to shift end-of-life care from acute care to other settings, funding has not followed services. The lack of full funding for care in other settings means that many people cannot afford to leave hospital or are forced into hospital to relieve the financial burden on their families, who face average costs of more than $24,000* per month in terms of travel, out-of-pocket expenses and time devoted to caregiving."

There has recently been some good news, at least in Ontario. The *Globe and Mail*** reported in April 2015 that the provincial government was planning on bumping the budget for home and community care by 5 percent in 2015, "but," it went on, "it still makes up a small fraction of overall health spending. The government is promising $750 million more for the sector over the next three years."

One of the reasons for the vast cost difference between home care and hospice, and hospital care is that treating patients at home allows the system to take advantage of free labour. Husbands, lovers, wives, or other relatives and friends give up work to take care of their dying loved ones. There is some relief for those who need to take a leave of absence from their job to care for someone, at least in Ontario. The government will pay EI to caregivers for eight weeks in any given six month period. It's something, but it hardly matches the loss of income. The Expert Group on Home & Community Care commented: "On average, in Canada, family caregivers provide about seven hours of help to family and friends for every two hours of professional care. If we expect family caregivers to continue to support and care for their loved one, we need to support them."

---

* D.N. Guerriere, B. Zagorski, K. Fassbender, et al, "Cost Variations in Ambulatory and Home-Based Palliative Care," *Palliative Medicine*, 2010, published online. This figure of $24,000 a month seems huge. However, the study's authors (who included, co-incidentally, Larry Librach) took into account not only lost work hours for caregivers, but also lost leisure time, and the potential costs to the health-care system if their care had to be replaced by a personal support worker.

** "Ontario Budget Continues Hard Line on Health Care in Bid to Tackle Deficit," *Globe and Mail*, April 23, 2015, www.theglobeandmail.com/news/national/ontario-budget-continues-hard-line-on-health-care-in-bid-to-tackle-deficit/article24094494.

"Obviously," Larry said, "hospital administrators would love to see more home-based care, because that saves them money. But the people that have to pay the physicians [to work in the community] don't put money in the pot, because they don't see the savings. It comes from a different pot. And nobody is willing to force that. The reality is than it can be quite expensive to keep somebody at home, but it's still cheaper that an ICU bed. For a hospital administrator it means that they can make their limited resources go farther. They may not see more patients, but they can make [the money] go farther and they don't have to make as many cuts. But I don't think there's anyone in the system that really wants to tackle the problem. How are you going to take away money from hospitals? You'll have people crying in the streets. When you look at what Ontarians want from health care the top two things are an emergency bed and a hospital bed when they need it. Anywhere between ten and fourteen on the list is home care.

"People aren't aware of the home-care system. They think it's charity. 'No, we don't need a nurse coming in.' Well, yes you do, you're taking gobs of opioids and you're getting weaker, you need an occupational therapist or physiotherapist to come in and make sure your house is okay if you want to stay at home. You need twenty-four-seven coverage. We might be able to find a physician for you, depending where you are in the city of Toronto. But in most parts of Canada you won't find that. So what do you do?

"People don't know anything about it, until they need it. And then when you do get it, it's ridiculous. They were supposed to send an occupational therapist in to see how we are doing. It's now been six weeks, we haven't seen hide nor hair of the occupational therapist. Oh well, we put in the request … we can only send out a physiotherapist once. Well, that's not helpful. Those are warts in the system that nobody wants to tackle. Health care in the community is in a terrible state, because we have become so hospital focused. If you're the executive director of a hospital you make a hell of a lot more money than an executive director of a home-care agency."

According to the Canadian Hospice Palliative Care Association's June 2010 policy brief, "Canadians will not receive high quality end-of-life care in all settings where they die until services in all these settings are funded equitably. Canada's health-care systems continue to fully fund only hospital and physician services. Long-term care services are only partially funded, and there are limits on the amount of home-care services that people receive. Hospice programs continue to rely on fund-raised dollars. Even the Victoria Hospice program, which is an integral part of its regional health authority, depends on fund raising to deliver what most would argue are essential end-of-life services. According to a recent study, the health-care system pays about seventy percent of the cost of end-of-life care — mainly related to hospital stays, while families pay twenty-seven percent and non-for-profit organizations about two percent."

The report concluded that "lack of funding also means that even high-functioning integrated programs do not have the resources they require to meet the growing demand for end-of-life care. They are currently not able to meet the needs of everyone in their catchment area who could benefit from their services. What will they do over the next ten years as the number of people dying and the demand for care increase?"

CHAPTER 9

Song

Summer 2013 was a particularly damp one in Toronto. And yet every time I made the subway journey to Larry's condo the sun shone out of a clear blue sky as I emerged from St. Clair West subway station, as it did on the morning of Victoria Day, May 20. Natalie came with me. She hadn't seen Larry since his retirement party.

I was pleased to see him up and about when we got to the condo. Faye had written the previous week to tell me his chemo on Thursday had been cancelled, because he hadn't been able to bounce back from the chemo the week before. He was using his cane and still moving slowly, but some of his old energy was back. His moustache was well groomed, the crease in his dark-blue trousers razor sharp, his button-down Oxford crisp. He led us into the sitting room and sat in the armchair, his back to the view of Cedarvale Park. We took the couch.

"I'm glad, because I was going to tell them I wasn't going to go in for the chemo anyway." He laid his hand on Natalie's forearm, adopted a confidential tone. "At least I'm able to walk a little bit now. After Phil left last week I was barely able to walk."

I held my hands up. "It wasn't anything I did."

His laugh was back too. "I'm just saying, nobody else did that to me. I used to have patients in the mafia. I don't anymore, so you're lucky." He turned serious. "So I'm using a cane now and I use a wheelchair when we're outside, but I was barely able to walk."

Larry asked Faye for his sippy cup. Faye asked Natalie if she'd like a drink too, but she declined. I, on the other hand, never turn down coffee. I turned the microphone on Larry, and asked the question that was becoming my regular opening. How had he been the previous week?

"I wasn't able to do anything last week. Literally lay in bed most of the time, felt sorry for myself. I'm not the type of person that gets immobilized. I didn't even have the energy to open a keyboard. So it was" — Larry adopted a sing-song voice — "a problem."

But at least things had settled down. His home-care nurse had been arranged and had visited, as had his palliative-care physician, David Kendal. "David has been absolutely amazing."

Natalie, who worked with David, cut in. "It's hard for him too."

"It is. But you know, he said to me, 'I want to continue learning from you, but on the other hand, you've got to pay attention to me, I'm the doctor.' So having him is a blessing. He's so steady."

There had been good news the previous week. Despite Larry's challenges with the chemo, his post-chemo lab results were in, and there were strong indications it was working. "They look at these tumour markers now, and one of them is the CA antigen." Tumours trigger an immune response in their host, because they produce antigens (usually proteins). Oncologists call these antigens tumour markers. By measuring the levels of these markers, oncologists can tell how active a tumour is. "My CA antigen went down by twenty-five percent with just two small doses of chemo. So that impressed my doctors. It certainly impressed David Warr." David was one of Larry's colleagues in the pain clinic. "He said I should have a wonderful weekend. Actually I had not a bad weekend. I'm starting to get some energy back. So there is some evidence that the chemo may work. At least to help me a little bit ..."

Larry caught himself mid-sentence. He was living in a bubble, and in this bubble everyone was hoping for a miracle. The bubble amplifies everything, magnifies any shred of hope, and good news is glommed onto ferociously. He was keenly aware of this, knew even this good news had to be put into its proper context: "But I'm not ... I mean I know what my story is, what the end point will be. But if I can add some quality of life to all that. If I can have some good days, like yesterday and probably today as well, well then at least I can see myself spending some more time with my grandkids."

His voice dropped again, as if he were imparting a secret, or telling a slightly off-colour joke: "I don't care about work anymore. I gave it up so easily. It's quite amazing, but even at that tribute luncheon, which was absolutely phenomenal, that set me on a course of saying I've got to do these things because I've got my family, and I've got myself to look after now." It was very explicitly part of his mission — the message to focus on your family and on the things that matter, and to pay less attention to the details, which seem to matter in the moment but don't. "If I can have that kind of effect on anybody, including my family, then there's been a success at least somewhere in there."

But there was a tension at work here, wasn't there? Here I was, recorder in front of him, stealing his time and energy. We had made his journey public. Wouldn't that impact his family? I'd no doubt these sessions were tiring. I was careful to limit them to no longer than an hour. I'd stopped our last meeting at the forty-five-minute mark because Larry was looking tired. And how could that not impact the time he spent with Faye? The time he spent with Judith, David, and his grandchildren. Was I robbing them of the best of him in these final few months? It worried me. Now was probably a good time to raise my concerns. "So why did you agree to go public with this, Larry? Most people would say just hide it and deal with it."

"I spent all my life trying to tell people it's okay to talk about dying and it's okay to talk about cancer. Why would I not want to talk about it now?"

I could think of any number of reasons. Because people often find the things they believe in theory are very much harder to live by in practice? Because everyone would understand if he said he just wanted to dedicate his last days to his wife and family, and not put himself though this? Because he obviously had limited energy, and every one of our sessions would drain him, at least a little? Because he'd already achieved so much and his legacy was already assured? Because he could give himself a pass? And a thousand other reasons, all of them good, that would have justified a withdrawal.

But it was clear Larry couldn't imagine why he wouldn't take this last opportunity. It was his last, best, teachable moment. For as hard as it is to teach patients to die well, it is far harder to live those precepts day by day as the clock ticks down to our own death. The principle of the thing is fine, but it quickens when we see it lived out.

"I know it's not the Orthodox Jewish way of dealing with it. But I want to be able to let people know. It's gone all across Canada and my friends in Europe and my friends down south. They all know about all of this. I've made no bones about the fact that I know my diagnosis."

As to the impact on his family, he didn't see it getting in the way. On the contrary, he believed it would help both him and his family. He wondered if it was perhaps the best legacy he could leave. He was touched by the tributes that still poured in. The memorial luncheon made a huge impact on him. It buoyed him, set him on a fair course for his final few months. But he also had no illusions about his legacy. He didn't expect memorials or statues. "I've always said there'll be a Larry Librach memorial urinal. I know I'll be forgotten. Why should I think I'll be any different than anyone else?"

Larry switched gears, as Larry would. It wasn't a symptom. It was just Larry. A bubble of thought rose up from somewhere in his subconscious and burst into the room. I was used to it by then; I'd known him long enough to ride these switches.

"Last week, I gotta tell you this, you know the kid's group Sharon, Lois and Bram?"

I shook my head, shrugged a little. Natalie laughed. "He's English."

Faye, who until now had pottered around in the kitchen and answered the continuous stream of phone calls, came to sit in on the conversation.

"Ahh, yes, he missed out on the cultural experience," Larry said. Without skipping a beat, he broke into song, as if this would somehow explain everything: "Skinnamarinky dinky do. I love you." I assumed this was a reference to some of Sharon, Lois and Bram's work, and not a sudden confession of previously suppressed emotion.

"They were big for years. We took our kids to see them. Faye is friends with Bram's sister-in-law and she spoke to Faye and arranged for them to come — at least Sharon and Bram, because Lois doesn't sing with them anymore. So they came last Thursday and did a little private concert for my grandchildren. As it turns out, Russell looked after Bram's wife when she was dying and Sharon's husband when he died. They were both on our program.

"So they did this incredible little concert downstairs in the condo's party room. There were seven kids and about twenty adults."

He leant back into his chair, a distant look in his eyes, clearly savouring the memory. "Those kinds of things are incredibly precious … I mean, I was in tears the whole time. But singing skinnamarinky dinky do," Larry turned to Faye, "you've been singing it in your head for about a week. Or … five little monkeys playing on a bed, one fell off and hit his head, took him to the doctor who said …"

"All right, Larry. We don't want to hear the whole thing," Faye said. She was a school principal and still retains the ability to send a finger of ice down even an adult's spine with a single glance. It was always their dynamic; Larry the court jester, Faye reigning him in when his ebullience threatened to break out too far.

I confess, I was surprised. My initial reaction being, why not let him go with it? He had little enough time left to him. Let him sing. But then I remembered they'd been together for over forty years. It wasn't a reflection on the state of their relationship. Or perhaps it was just that. Their relationship was standing up. This was their way and it was unchanged by Larry's diagnosis. It was comforting; some habits are too deeply threaded to be easily displaced, even by something as grave as mortal illness.

Larry picked up the conversation as if nothing had happened. "So anyway, it was incredible. My three-year-old grandson sang all the words to the songs, and the girls took part. We had some pizza afterward. It was a quite amazing afternoon. Hopefully it will stick in my grandkids' heads, and their parents' heads too."

Speaking of memories reminded Larry of the memory boxes he was putting together for his grandkids. "I'm doing some of the things I told patients to do."

The idea was to fill the boxes with things to celebrate and memorialize the special events in the childhoods and adolescent lives of his grandkids, and provide some mementos of Larry. It had become something of an obsession, a project that he was determined to finish.

Carrie, the volunteer from Hospice Toronto who helped Larry put the memory boxes together, has a background in fine arts. She is also a qualified arts therapist. "She seems younger than young," Larry said. "She came in and we started talking and I got the sense that she hasn't done this before. Well, she's in her early twenties, so she doesn't have a lot of experience. So she was really looking forward to this and we're trying to sort out what could be in them. You don't want to do too much, and I wanted to do something I could work on this week. I've got a few things I have to put together, but who gets involved in this? Is it just my task, do we involve my grandkids?

"This will be my gift to them. I'm not worried they're going to forget me. I want them, at times in their lives that are important, to remember who they are, rather than who I am. I've started doing the letters I'm putting in for each of them. They have to be different enough, but also contain some of the same messages. The girls will receive them for their bat mitzvahs: so Ella's is in two years and Jessie's is two years after that. Last week, even in the midst of feeling absolutely shitty, I went to Yorkdale and I bought the girls each a piece of jewellery for their bat mitzvahs. And then for the little guy, Finn, I mean he's only three. We're getting an oil painting of him in his hockey outfit. Just his parka with his hockey stick. A friend of ours does oil paintings from photos, so that will be his first gift. We figure he'll get it when he starts grade one." Larry dropped his voice half an octave, a habit he had when joking. "He's a little more difficult to buy jewellery for. And then at his bar mitzvah, so that's another ten years down the road, he'll get a letter. And when the girls finish school and Finn finishes high school we've put aside some Israeli bonds they'll be able to use to travel to Israel, or to travel anywhere ... just some travel money. After high school kids should get out there and not just prepare for university or whatever. Have some fun.

"Carrie and I are just trying to look at the formatting: do you have a big box with little boxes inside? Do you have a key on the box, which I think is always the best for kids because they're inquisitive little souls.

"And then, what is the timetable for this? If you make it long will it be too long? If short, too short? And then who has responsibility? Because we're putting bonds inside the parents will have some responsibility for keeping them current. They'll come due before the kids get them so they'll have to be renewed. Carrie's coming back on Monday with some ideas about what the boxes should look like, but it's all new to her, I have more experience than she does and I can't tell you that I have a lot of experience. I certainly have zero artistic talent."

The boxes are another of reminder, of course. Most things are now. What the scholars of medieval Europe called a *memento mori* ("remember that you have to die"). In medieval Europe philosophers believed that if we are to learn to cope with the notion of death, we should spend our lives reflecting on it. The notion infuses the art and literature of the period. It's almost the polar opposite of our modern attitude toward death, which is to avert our gaze, or if someone raises the subject to quickly change it.

It was past time to leave and let Larry rest, but his strength and energy was obviously bouncing back, because he wouldn't let us leave without booking another meeting for later in the week. Faye marked it on the calendar, May 24, and we said our goodbyes. The next day I transferred the audio of the interview into an audio editor and isolated Larry singing "Skinnamarinky." Natalie wanted to take it into work to cheer everyone up. And it did. It was so typically Larry.

CHAPTER 10

Burden

That week was a busy one for Larry. On Thursday he recorded an interview about his cancer journey with the Canadian Partnership Against Cancer (CPAC) for their *The Truth of It* video series. *The Truth of It* interviews Canadians who have been diagnosed with cancer and asks them to share their story so others can learn from their experience. On Friday, Rick Firth, board executive at the Canadian Hospice Palliative Care Association (CHPCA), was due to call in to drop off the plaque for the Balfour Mount Champion Award, which Larry had been awarded in April.

We wouldn't have our normal hour, but it hardly mattered. Larry was clearly bouncing back from the chemo, and was relishing his regained energy. He didn't rule out going back on the chemo completely, but it seemed to me he'd take some convincing. I'd never seen him so insistent.

I knew we wouldn't have long to talk, so I focused our discussion on a topic that had been playing on my mind for the past several days. We'd talked about how crucial it is to communicate with family and loved ones, tell them how you're feeling. To be truthful, and not to withhold information. It's something Larry mentioned the first time I visited. A weakness, he'd discovered, even he was prone to. I'd salted it away, meaning to ask him to expand on it.

"You said you've found yourself falling into the same patterns and behaviours you've seen in other people when they're sick. You'd noticed you pushed Faye and the family away, creating an emotional distance.

You caught yourself and talked yourself out of it. But it's interesting that even you, a seasoned palliative-care physician, fell foul of this impulse."

"That's part of the conversation Anne and I are having." Anne Langlois was a former colleague of Larry's at the Latner Centre. "How much do you let go, knowing the person who is receiving the information may be hurt by it? But the person at the other end may actually want to hear that information."

For Larry this attitude, this way of thinking, arises from the patient's anxiety. We create for ourselves these chimeras of the imagination and they dominate our thoughts. The monster tells us we're a burden and we believe it. It tells us we're useless, no longer needed, part of the past; a useless, used up, and diseased body about to become a cadaver.

"David Kendal always catches me with that word, *burden*, because we use it all the time. You know, 'I don't want to be a burden to my family.' We often say the reason for admission to hospice is because the patient doesn't want to be a burden to their family. Assisted death, same thing, 'Don't want to be a burden to my family.' Well, what does that actually mean? If you've got a strong enough family and you've got coping mechanisms and you've coped with crises before, you have an interdependency that's really important for both sides of the equation." Larry paused, brought the discussion back to his own situation, his own disease, his own family. "So it's important for Faye and for my kids to know how I'm feeling. But it may not be as important for my grandkids to know." Not that you should shield them from knowing you're ill. Larry had always been very clear about this. The instinct to protect our children from the realities of the situation will certainly have negative repercussions later on, and may cause immediate problems. Children are far more perceptive than we give them credit for. They probably know more about the situation than the adults around them would like to believe. Still, Larry said, they don't need to know every detail; there has to be "some protectiveness there."

"And you need to share the things that are important. If you are having a down day people will see that. Because when you keep things inside, what you see happening is people become depressed. They become irritable. They become angry. They become more demanding. They actually become more of a burden and they withdraw emotionally. There's no hugging, there's no kissing, there's a sense of trying to protect [their families by not] being a burden. At the same time they are becoming more of a burden."

It was tempting to ask, "Is that it?" As if truth, honesty, and openness couldn't possibly be enough. Isn't the pattern too deeply woven into our natures? I recognized the pattern, remember Sally telling me that John withdrew when he was told his cancer was terminal. His conversation collapsed. Questions about her daughters, their jobs, their lives, dried up. He'd respond to her questions, when she asked them, but his answers were monosyllabic, more grunts than answers. Of course, the tracheotomy didn't help. It was another barrier to communication. One that John no longer wanted to surmount.

I'm convinced John believed he acted with the best of intentions. He cut us loose so he wouldn't drag us down with him, like a mountaineer who cuts his line rather than pull his friends from the rock face. Still, despite the fact that I'd witnessed the damage this withdrawal can do first-hand, I wanted a more complex solution to the problem from Larry than simply "communicate." Something perhaps involving complex instrumentation or brain surgery. Could this really be how we break the pattern? Larry insisted it was. And although it sounds simple, that doesn't make it easy.

"What David Kendal said to me, and what I've said to patients over the years, is this withdrawal doesn't work. You fall into the trap, think you're a burden and that maybe it would be better just to push off and be admitted to hospital, or to not talk about it and cry yourself to sleep.... That's all fine, but it doesn't work. It doesn't protect you and it doesn't relieve their burden."

There's another dimension to this too: the burden the patient has to carry. Larry had first-hand experience of this. During his ordeal with jaundice he became increasingly frustrated with the system, his doctors, his inability to control events and their outcome. This sudden helplessness is frightening as well as frustrating, but patients typically suffer it in silence, withdrawing, holding the turmoil in.

"If you withdraw, you increase your burden on yourself. Talking is important. The people that can't talk about it really, really suffer. I've seen that over the years. The people who can't talk about what's going on and their frustrations really suffer. And the system is frustrating. But all systems are frustrating. When you find a perfect system, let" — Larry paused briefly, because he remembered this ends "let me know," which didn't quite work anymore, given his diagnosis — "Let somebody know."

But isn't there also a cultural dimension to this? Larry's already said this open attitude he promoted is not exactly the way of Jewish orthodoxy. Practising in Toronto, one of the most culturally diverse cities in the world, surely must have given him a unique perspective on the cultural spectrum?

Larry rubbed the end of his nose with his knuckle. It was something I'd noticed before — a little physical tic you begin to see when you spend long enough with a person. He dragged one of his anecdotes up out of deep memory.

"I had this one patient, she was Portuguese. And she was dying. Getting quite close to death. And the family was really quite distraught. They called me into the living room when I arrived. This was before I'd even been in to see her. And they said, 'We know she's coming to the end, we know she's dying. But please don't tell her.' So then they usher me into her room, and the curtains are drawn, and there are candles burning. And there were women, professional mutes, standing around the bed." The use of mutes — generally women, who are paid to mourn a dying or dead loved one — is a forgotten tradition, even in Europe, but they are still occasionally used by some more traditionally minded families. "She tells me she wants to speak to me alone. She waves the family out. She was quite weak, but she still had the strength for that. She gestures to me to move closer, and she says: 'Doctor, I know I'm dying, but please don't tell my family.'"

He leant forward for his sippy cup. "So, yes, it's an issue for sure, and not talking about things really increases your burden. There are cultures that don't allow you to talk, but there's always somebody in a family you can talk to. There's always some way you can unburden yourself. But unburdening myself to my fourth cousin is not the same as unburdening to Faye. Unburdening to my rabbi is not the same as unburdening to my spouse, or my daughter."

"So, as a physician, how did you cut through that?"

"Just by pointing out that it's a burden of love. It's a burden for families to share, not a burden individuals need to bear alone. We defend our family together, we promote our family together, we grow together. And it's that togetherness that protects you from the burden. People accept the burden. It's part of the love. There's always going to be a burden to love."

I wondered what he meant by that? "A burden to love?" It's hardly what we expect of love, hardly what we imagine it to be: a burden.

"Once you get married you accept the burden that you are now two people and that has to be considered in whatever you do. If you have a family, then there's three or four. There's extended family, brothers, and sisters that have to be dealt with. But if you don't share that together there was no point in getting married. And life is never a straight line. Things change. When you first get married it's very different to your life three or four years later, and that's hugely different to your life forty years later. But the love, that's still core. I used to ask families, what do you mean by burden? What's the burden? And they'd answer, well, it's the physical burden of looking after someone who's sick. So I'd tell them that's why we are here to help you. We'll help as much as we can with the physical burden. We can't take it all away, but we'll help. So then they'd say, well, it's watching him suffer. Or if I was talking to the patient, it's them watching me suffer. But you do that. You want to help. And so I usually took them back to a time where they coped with another crisis and said, how did you get through that? How did you manage that? That was a burden at that time, and look, you managed that. This is the final burden. But afterward, that burden pays off because you've helped somebody. You've reduced some of your own suffering in that way too because things were more open and your grief will have been much less. And at the end of it you will have a sense of satisfaction. The thing about home palliative care that's very different than you see in hospitals is a sense of satisfaction that families have in providing home care. Now, we don't recognize that. We don't support them enough and give them enough psychosocial support. The system is crazy that way."

Ahh, the system. The way we've medicalized death, swept it out of sight into clinically controlled environments, ignoring the human dimension, the gut shreddingness of the emotions that tear into us at such a time. But although we imagine it that way, the reality is surprising. "When I first went into home palliative care, I expected I would go to pronounce somebody dead and there'd be rending of clothes and sackcloth and ashes and crying all over." I couldn't help but smile as Larry demonstrated for me by flailing his arms around his head, his sudden animation startling, driving me back into the safe embrace of the armchair. "But more often than not there was just a simple peace in the family. There were some tears. You'd go in and say hello to the family, you'd check the patient out, because everybody wants to make sure the patient's dead so you have to at least do the pulse, look at the pupils, are they fixed and dilated, close the eyes, touch the patient. I think it's very important that physicians, when they pronounce somebody, touch the patient and show people it's okay to touch somebody who is dead. There's nothing nasty about it. But then you go into the kitchen and they would often present you with a glass of Scotch or something. Or a tea, or cookie, and there would be, as well as the tears, some laughter. 'Well, mom would have liked this, all of us standing around here.' Or there would be that pathos. Which is very different than what you see in a sterile environment like a hospital. Hospices are different and palliative-care units. But it's that sense of satisfaction they had in looking after their loved one."

Larry was careful to make sure they understood the emotional heft of what they'd done. He knew they would be confused and in shock. And there's so much to do when somebody dies, a funeral to arrange, bank accounts to close, things to dispose of; an avalanche of details. "But I would encourage them to stop for a moment, to realize what an important thing they have done. Not only for the patient, but also for themselves. Because they now know what dying is like and we are all going to have to face that. Now they can teach their children. So when people are worrying about burdens I say yes, it is a burden. But it's a burden you accept because you are family. And yes, if it becomes too burdensome we will need to look at ways of supporting you and maybe a palliative unit, but that's not failure."

It's easy to underestimate the traumas that caregivers experience. The emotional and physical impact of caring for a dying loved one, the sheer exhaustion of it. Many, probably most, try to cover it up, to wear their bravest face when they're in the presence of the dying, but it's impossible to hide. Most dying people understand their caregiver's limits are being tested, which adds to the weight of the guilt and helplessness they feel themselves. It's the most common problem people face when they're dying, Larry said. "And yet a hundred years ago it wasn't that way, because you expected to maintain the burden. There were no hospitals. You expected to stay home and have granny at home until she died." He's right, of course. We moved death out of the home in the twentieth century. According to Statistics Canada, almost 65 percent of deaths in Canada take place in hospital. So we've tidied death away in sanitized, sterile environments that give us the illusion we're controlling it. Or worse, prevent us from needing the illusion at all anymore. We've created a new illusion, that death is not all around us all the time. That it's diminishingly rare. I'm sixty years old and I've never seen a dead body. Both my parents and all of my grandparents are dead, but I never saw them after their death.

But here we were again, talking about the system. I was interested in Larry. "So what was it exactly that you caught yourself doing, that you'd seen your patients doing through the years?" I asked.

"I avoided conversations when I felt hurt. And there were several times when I wanted just to scream out and I didn't do it because I didn't want my family to be involved. Yet I needed the support at the time, particularly around those procedures, you know." He was referring to the operations on his bile duct, and the fiascos that surrounded them. "I just wanted to punch somebody out! Even the nurses, when I think back, I had very little nursing support in the palliative-care unit. That's because the budget's been cut and all. There was only one nurse, the nurse in charge, who actually sat down one day and asked me how I was, and how was my pain, did I have any breakthrough pain? Did I have a bowel movement? This is your blood pressure and here are your new sheets and your robe. But there were times when I knew that I needed help and I didn't ask for it. Being at home, I've been a lot freer with asking for help with Faye."

That's part of it then, a big part. Just being heard, being cared for. But there's something else too: this belief that it's weak to show our feelings when we're overwhelmed. To be stoic in the face of pain and suffering is to be strong. It's generations-deep, this attitude: be a man, take your medicine, stand tall, stiff upper lip, smile in the face of adversity. Larry learned to swim against the tide of such advice, and he said it did him a world of good.

"I just needed that support at the time. So I let it all hang out and I felt much better for it. I was able to carry on. If I had left it inside it would've eaten away until it came out and then it might come out in anger. It often does. Anger toward the health-care providers ... that damn doctor he doesn't tell me things and he doesn't do this ... and I know he's keeping things back and they don't care about me, I'm just a number.... You see this all the time, just blame the system. Sometimes the system has to be blamed but the system also has to listen to these complaints and has to be aware of the conflicts. You can't shy away from them."

And if it's true that there's no perfect system, no perfect patient, it must be equally true there's no perfect family.

"Faye and I always joke about that, you know, it's your crazy family, nobody is crazy on my side of the family and we look at each other and just laugh."

What you may not anticipate is dependency. It's another of our society's strongest dogmas, to cherish and preserve our independence. No doubt this is linked to the "don't be a burden" doctrine, but it's also tied to pride, to our sense of self. The I who is master of my own destiny, standing up for myself, having and exercising choice. It's arguably the best thing about growing up. We determine our own fate. We don't have to rely on anyone else for anything.

"Becoming dependent was one of my big fears," Larry said. "And I am dependent on people now. There's no question about it. I'm dependent on the nurse to give me my injections, because my hands are so shaky I couldn't give them to myself. I'm dependent on my kids to help support me. Faye, of course, but other family members, friends, all are vitally important. They don't mind doing it. I know that as I get sicker I will call on them to do a little bit more, and that's what I will need. I need people to take me to chemo. I need people to take me for blood tests, because I can't do it. I can't take the subway. I can't drive. It's a time for me to reach out to people as well. You can't maintain total independence. When I saw patients trying to do that, they lost. They put themselves into safety problems. Then they put themselves into 'damn it all' and anger and unresolved conflict. But fortunately, almost all of us can call on family. Of course, you have to define family in a looser way ... the group of people you call on for support, because it may not be your core family. It may be a really good friend, a fourth cousin, your neighbour next door. I used to see that all the time. It could be hospice volunteers that become part of the family. There's always family that can help out."

I lean forward, pick up the coffee mug, and fold my hands around it. Larry's jolted me out of the present, brought my younger brother Barrie to mind. A gay man who saw many of his friends suffer and die in the early years of the AIDS epidemic in the early to mid-eighties. None of us, his brothers and sisters, knew what Barrie went through during those years. We still don't. He doesn't speak of it. But it's clear to all of us the trauma of watching so many friends die tragic and horrible deaths has left its mark. For a several years Barrie withdrew from the family, feeling our worlds were so different we couldn't understand him or his experience. Feeling, no doubt, that his true family were his friends. It's understandable: they felt besieged, in a fight with a virus that hadn't even been identified at that point.

Many of Barrie's friends had been disowned by their families, and although he wasn't, I think we all understood how such traumas would open up a gulf between Barrie and the rest of us. During those days most of us understood why Barrie felt that his true family were the people fighting AIDS on the front line.

"I know what you're talking about," I said. "It doesn't have to be a family, it can be a community. I'm thinking of the gay community during the AIDS epidemic."

"Oh yeah, and I saw that at the time ... that was probably the most stressful palliative-care experience I had. Our patient load was twenty to forty percent HIV patients. Frank Ferris," the physician with whom Larry co-founded the Temmy Latner Centre, "and I had gotten into this and didn't even realize what was happening." These were the very early days of palliative care in Canada. Frank and Larry had not long set up the service that was to become the Latner Centre, just at the time when AIDS was cutting a swath through Toronto's gay community. "We were pronouncing ten people a day, watching these guys die horrible deaths. But then seeing also the caring of the families ... not only their partners, but their club groups. The way they would form care teams and would care for each other. It was spiritually uplifting, but at the same time watching their agony: having pneumocystis pneumonia and having diarrhea until their guts were pouring out, and dying of diarrhea and so wasted that you could pick them up. They were thirty and forty pounds, literally skin and bones. That was the most stressful part of palliative care that we went through. It was just awful, it was … we were saints at that time. I mean nobody else was providing care at home. There was a primary HIV group that we taught about palliative care, but we were often sharing care. There were some amazing physicians, many of them gay themselves, but a lot of them not. The communities they represented were their surrogate families. It was amazing to see it.

"Frank Ferris was gay so … big deal…. It was Frank who set me on the path of real acceptance, so it didn't bother me to walk into alternative living habits and I didn't care about their sexual habits. It didn't make any difference. I was there for their suffering and to support their families and to support the burden of care on these young men, watching as they watched friend after friend after friend die."

My conversation with Larry about the way AIDS decimated a generation of young gay men had stirred another memory, of Barrie's reaction when he visited John in hospital.

Sally was devastated by the change she saw in John, and she prepared Barrie for a similar shock. However, Barrie hardly seemed to be affected by John's condition. He told Sally that John hadn't looked as bad as he'd expected.

I wasn't there that day, but Sally called me a few days later. She worried that she'd exaggerated the gravity of John's condition. She was upset and confused, anxious for me to see John for myself, to find out what I felt.

We wondered out loud if Barrie's experiences with AIDS had hardened him.

The truth, as it turned out, was a little more complex. Barrie had been changed by his experiences with AIDS, but not in the way we believed. He was careful to present a positive, optimistic face to John. He'd seen friends recover against similar odds. It wasn't, he felt, a time to give up, which demonstrates, if nothing else, how easy it is to misinterpret the words and actions of those around us, especially in the midst of grief.

That is not to say that people don't get hardened in extreme conditions. "You can become very hardened," Larry said. "The people who became very hardened were some of the HIV-specialist physicians. They were often very critical of their clients behind their back."

We were coming to the end of our hour, and though Larry still showed no signs of flagging, Rick Firth would be arriving any minute. I also didn't want to push Larry too hard, so I asked a final question before leaving. "How do you go about talking to the family about your fears and your feelings? How do you achieve that openness?"

"You make sure you've had those conversations at some point in the past. Because there's always time for crucial conversations with family. It's really important not to keep secrets in families, especially about illness. Faye's family has done that for years." It's a common reaction to bad news, Larry said: "Don't tell anybody they have diabetes, or this or that condition.' You don't have to do that. You need to let people know and you need to be able to have advanced-care-planning conversations, for instance, when you're healthy, not when you're lying in a critical-care unit and somebody has to make decisions for you at a time when you can't help yourself."

It's a vital point, and one people rarely think about until it's almost too late. Because if you leave the conversation too late your loved ones may be called upon in a crisis to make decisions on your behalf, and have to guess what you might really want. If you go into cardiac arrest, should you be given CPR? Should you be kept alive at any cost? Even if you're in a total vegetative state? This requires some thought, because it's not just a binary decision: to revive you or not. The real question is what is your minimum tolerable quality of life? Would you want to live if you couldn't walk? If you were totally paralyzed? If you were brain damaged?

"So I think the idea is to practise decision-making in this way and to keep it open and allowed. Every family suffers deaths over a period of time, so talk about it. Whether it's Uncle Joe or Cousin Theresa or whatever, you can talk about it openly, let your kids go to the funerals. Let them see the mourning. They can be at wakes or Shivas. They can see grief. When somebody important dies discuss it."

I wasn't sure what Larry meant by someone important. Someone important in the family, or someone important in the wider world? A star, a big name who can be used to start the conversation? "Someone famous, but also make it clear that ordinary people's lives have meaning and purpose. I like that sometimes the back page of the *Globe* runs obituaries of normal people. I think it really helps people understand ordinary lives can have meaning and purpose.

"The other thing to think about is your own spirituality. There's a spirituality that's not religion. Whether you believe in religion or not, you can just sit there on the dock, look out with your kids, and listen to the waves wave. Listen to thunder, feel the wind in your face, look out on the greenery, the snow. Look at the stars. Be with your family so that they aren't afraid when disasters happen.

"It's a sense of connection with the universality of things and people. Not enough people stop to enjoy the world, to enjoy life. Whether you're fishing or you're at the theatre, whatever you're doing. And knowing that it will come to an end. That's important too.

"That's my spirituality. Do I believe there's a God up there waving fingers at us individually, who knows exactly what I'm thinking every moment of every day? I think he's got too important a job to do that.

"But go back to your religion, if that's what you've grown up on and if that's where you find solace. I find solace in Jewish music, I find solace in some of the prayers, ordinary prayers, the walk through the valley of the shadow of death. People are surprised to learn the Psalms are Jewish not Christian.

"When I used to advise people I said don't ignore that part of your life. You can spend a lot of time thinking, 'Why is God doing this to me?' But you can find your own meaning in purpose in your life. That's your spirituality too. Look at your grandkids. Look at what you've done, what you've made. You know they won't survive, more than a few years anyway. Nobody remembers who Timothy Eaton was anymore; they took his statue down because people were defacing it. They didn't know who he was.

"People have always tried to create legacies for themselves, tried to conquer the world. But Alexander the Great died, Genghis Khan died, all the dynasties in China died, at great cost to human life. Napoleon died, and is now remembered as a pastry or a brandy. For me, my legacy is those boxes I'm doing. My legacy is some of the things people have told me that I've helped them create themselves. There's the Latner Centre, for as long as that lasts, but in ten years who's Librach? But that's okay. It doesn't bother me that I may be forgotten, because eventually even my relatives will forget me. There will be a limited memory two hundred years from now. But that's okay. I feel I've lived a full life."

There was a knock on the condo's door. Faye went to answer it, and called from the hall. Rick had arrived to present Larry with his award. I was shanghaied into the role of photographer for the presentation. As Larry said, "You have to be dying around here to get some recognition."

We made tentative plans to meet again the following week. Larry was still insistent he wasn't going back to chemo. But then, early the following Thursday I heard on the Latner Centre grapevine he was at Princess Margaret taking his chemo. I knew I would ask him why the next time we met, but I suspected I already knew the answer.

There's one barely visible aspect of The Burden. Call it compliance in the hope of a reprieve. Call it magical thinking. Call it what you will, it takes its shape and form from our joint histories, and from the narratives of success and failure we've been taught since we were children. It is what patients do for their families and loved ones. They attempt to eat, even if the chemo has left them nauseous. They take the tests, even if the results show nothing more than what they already knew. They attempt to exercise, even though they are impossibly tired. They take the chemo, because who knows? They may be the one in a hundred or a thousand whom it saves. They try to remain cheerful and optimistic.

Our experience of life has conditioned us to believe in our sovereign ability to direct outcomes by our responses to life's challenges. And it works, in the main. Until we hit something that's impervious to our choices and our actions. Something like a fatal tumour. In the face of that threat a sunny disposition and a positive outlook are about as much use as an umbrella in a hurricane.

But patients fear that if they fail to remain positive the beast Burden will turn the ratchet one more notch on their family and friends, adding torture to torture.

CHAPTER 11

Hospice

When I first visited John in hospital in April 2010 it was hard to understand the words he huffed through his trach tube, but he was alert, his mind still sharp. He understood his prognosis. He knew he was dying, but he was insistent that he wanted to go home.

Over the next few weeks he continued to beg and cajole my sisters Sally and Julie about going home whenever he spoke with them. But his campaign went nowhere. He was assigned a Macmillan nurse — a nurse specializing in the care of cancer patients — and a social worker. Sally told me both her and Julie tried a number of times to speak with the Macmillan nurse. I believe she was probably understating her efforts. I've witnessed her fierce tenacity myself. She's a bulldog when she's roused. But the Macmillan nurse was never available when she called and never returned her calls. Still, Sally pressed the hospital staff and John's social worker about home care. She was told John needed round-the-clock care, which couldn't be provided at home. But the social worker suggested another option: Marie Curie Nurses. The Marie Curie Cancer Care charity provides round-the-clock nursing support for terminal patients at home and in its hospices. There were two problems with this option: there was a shortage of nurses in the Oldham area and John needed twenty-four-hour care, which could not be reliably guaranteed. But he clearly couldn't stay in hospital, taking up a valuable bed, a bed needed for the critically ill, not the chronically ill.

Finally, in mid-April, Sally and Julie's two-pronged assault yielded a result. John's social worker told them she was looking for a place in a long-term care home, not a hospice, as "Hospice places are for those at the end of their life." I was baffled. His tumour was inoperable. It had reduced him to little more than a skeleton. John was clearly at the end of his life. This conversation took place on April 14, 2010. He died scarcely three months later. Hospice was clearly the best place for him. I interpreted the decision as a tacit admission that there were no hospice spaces available. We've never had an explanation for this inexplicable decision.

Natalie and I weren't the only ones who were confused by the decision. "I was flummoxed," Sally said. When her mother-in-law had been admitted to a hospice twenty-four years previously she'd been in much better shape than John. "She was allowed to go home at weekends if she wanted to. It didn't make sense to me to put him in a home, only to have to refer him on to a hospice for end-of-life care. How long would that take? Would it even be possible?"

It took over six weeks to find John a care home and get him moved. By that time I'd given up any expectation of hospice care. John's social worker told Sally the reason for the six-week delay: the carers in the care home had to be trained to maintain John's feeding bag before he could be moved. Also, he needed a new Macmillan nurse, to replace the elusive Macmillan nurse at the hospital. Macmillan nurses who are attached to specific hospitals don't work in the community. "I couldn't understand why there wasn't a smoother transition from the hospital's Macmillan nurse to the external Macmillan nurse," Sally said. "They could share case notes and records. Surely that would make more sense?"

John clung on through April and May. He spent those months in the same hospital bed, staring out of the same window at the same narrow sliver of wall. During that time his condition worsened considerably. Sally said he was less alert, more withdrawn. John was finally found a place in a long-term care facility in May and was moved there in early June.

I learned about John's long-term care facility from an email my brother Stephen circulated to all my siblings. "It's purpose built and is clean and modern. The staff seems to be competent and caring, but there's a security code on the front door as the home also cares for the less mentally able." Stephen didn't tell me at the time, but I learned later that he was "confused" about the care worker's choice of home, because when he checked out the home's website it listed their specialty as dementia care.

But he "accepted that John's care worker had investigated and decided this was best suited to his needs."

A sanitizing euphemism that hardly prepared us for the reality — long-term care facilities are filled with human wreckage.

I didn't expect to see John alive again after I walked away from his hospital bed in April. And had it not been for the death of Natalie's grandmother in late June I wouldn't have done. Marge had low-grade leukemia, but that wasn't what killed her. She was just old, tired. Natalie's mother paid for Natalie and her sister Ingrid to fly to the U.K. for the funeral. It was another last chance to see John. I booked myself a flight.

We stayed with Natalie's aunt in Hereford, attended her grandmother's funeral a few days after arriving, and made plans to get to Manchester. There's a direct train service between Hereford and Manchester. Happily, this was the same train my mother's stylish and spry octogenarian younger sister — the only eighty-year-old I know who not only knows how to pronounce *quinoa*, but who actually eats it — caught from her home in Swansea. Freda met us on the train. Natalie and Freda chatted like old friends, arranging for Freda to use our Toronto condo as a staging post on future visits to her daughter, my cousin Suzie. Freda had slowed down in her eighties, and found the journey from the U.K. to visit Suzie in San Diego a little taxing.

Sally took the train from London and met us at Manchester's Piccadilly station. To keep things simple we stayed in a Travelodge in Oldham.

It was a fifteen-minute taxi ride the next morning from the Travelodge to John's long-term care home. It was another murky Manchester day. Grimy buildings flashing past the taxi's windows. Neglect and disrepair endemic, poverty visible, not just on the faces of pedestrians. It's ground into the brickwork of the Victorian buildings, a legacy of the wealth and prosperity of Manchester's industrial past. Now long past. A blackened patina that has worked its way into the nooks and crannies of the stone.

Past banks of shops, their metal shutters rolled down. Red-brick, two-storey terrace after terrace after terrace. *To Let* signs. Coiled barbed wire along the tops of walls. An Aldi. A Tesco. Even the windows to the steeple of St. John's the Evangelist boarded up. And as we drew closer to our destination, the new PVC doors and satellite dishes on the homes gave way to the previous generation's attempts at gentrification: Georgian-style doors in fake hardwood, the varnish peeled away, only the stain remaining in patches where it clung on longest. Tandoori houses. Chinese takeaways. Fish-and-chip shops.

We turned left. There was a house on the corner, painted white, its windows covered by solid sheets of metal painted British racing green. There was no signage, but it looked like another abandoned pub. The area was littered with them. Looks of hopelessness, or was it just crushing boredom, on the faces of passing strangers. Flimsy plastic shopping bags strained to contain cheap groceries, hung from the handles of a stroller. So heavy the child sitting in it was the only thing that kept its wheels on the ground. The mother, hair tied back from her face with elastic, no lippy or slap, her mouth a hyphen, hurried across the driveway as our taxi turned in, as fast as possible given her burdens.

The long-term care home itself. Lawns, tidy and well tended. A metal fence around the car park, seven feet tall. New and well-maintained.

Sally punched in the security code, turned the handle, and leant on the door. It buzzed and swung open under her weight. They lock the residents in, the mentally unstable ones at least. It's a long-term care home after all, not a hospice. The entranceway was obviously designed to be welcoming, cheerful. Celebrity magazines scattered enticingly on melamine coffee tables, fresh flowers in vases. But the cloying floral odour seemed too strong to be coming from the flowers, more like a scented candle or aromatherapy. Taupe and wheatmeal, the colours like nut milk and light rice. The colour of non-choice. A neutral colour. Neutered. Genderless.

We climbed the stairs, the four of us. It was tropically hot on the first floor, as if the staff were engaged in a delicate botanical operation, cultivating rare orchids. Perhaps the kind that only flower for a day. A curious thought to strike me as we made our way down the wheaty-walled corridors toward the light oak door of John's room. Our progress marked by the sound of our shoes on the tacky vinyl flooring, a sound a little like someone in the far distance tearing strips off a roll of adhesive tape.

We knocked, entered.

John lay on his bed in hospital robe and boxers. His giant flat-panel TV stood on a dresser on the other side of his bed, facing us. It dominated the room. Some variety of game show was playing, but John was asleep. Sally reached for the remote resting on top of the sheets, fumbled with it for a second, killed the sound, but left the TV on, flashing images of consumer heaven at us from across the narrow room.

John looked no worse than he had in hospital, but no better. He was tidier at least. His hair and beard a little better groomed. They'd been feeding him via a tube to his stomach, in an attempt to help him put on weight, but the fifty pounds he had lost were gone forever.

We settled in to wait for him to wake up. There was only one chair, which Freda took. Natalie, Sally, and I stood at the foot of the bed. Somewhere outside there was a crash. It sounded like a tray falling. Glasses breaking, perhaps. I opened the door and peered out. The home's communal lounge was across the hall and down the corridor a little. Someone was shouting. It may have been profanities, it was difficult to tell, because the words were slurred and uncertain. More moan and yowl than human speech. Someone, a staff member I judged, from the scrubs-style uniform, bustled past. "No need to worry." She smiled at me as she hurried past. "He's harmless. Just loud."

John's adopted daughter, Shirley, arrived with a friend. Until his admission to hospital in April, John had been Shirley's caregiver, shopping, cleaning, whatever she needed. A brain tumour had left her disabled, and John's help made it easier for her to cope with the demands of everyday life. Shirley and her friend had travelled by bus from their home in Oldham — had to change buses twice. We chatted a little. The journey up. The weather. "Cold for the time of year, isn't it? Miserable?"

John stirred, seemed to wake a little. Normally Sally would have stooped to kiss him, but we'd been warned by one of the staff that there should be no kissing. We might pass on an infection to him. It could be fatal. Danger lurked too in the cellophane bags of boiled sweets people had been bringing him. They had also been banned. Choking hazards, apparently.

So instead of kissing we shook hands. Shirley dug into her handbag. She'd brought John some cards from Phyllis's other children and his grandkids, and two helium-filled balloons. The metallic kind. HAPPY BIRTHDAY printed optimistically over their shiny silver faces. John's sixty-third birthday was in four days, July 6. She spoke loud and slow, to be certain he had understood. Repeated herself to drive it past the fog and confusion. Make it lodge there in the solid part of him that we were all sure was still in there somewhere. We saw it in glimpses when the fog cleared. But much less often than in April. In April he'd still had that mischievous spark that was undeniably John. That had gone.

At one point the conversation flagged. There was nothing more to be said about the rotten weather, the bus schedule, or the train journey, and we all cast around for similarly pale and flaccid topics of conversation. And speaking of pale and flaccid, John, who had barely been with us at all these past fifteen minutes, stirred on the bed. He appeared to be trying to insinuate a long, bony forefinger into the fly of his boxers. He was tentative at first, as though whatever was in there might be frightened away by sudden movement or the use of excessive force.

It called to my mind an image from my childhood: my grandmother, teasing a winkle from its shell with a pin. And I recalled, with a certain relish for the irony, that her polite, parlour euphemism for my penis was "winkle."

Then, with an almost triumphal flourish, he produced the pale and flaccid organ that had been the object of his probing finger. It must have been fifty years since I had last seen it, very likely during one of our "who can pee the highest" contests, which took place in the communal urinals at the holiday camps we visited in the summers of my childhood. John, legs akimbo, to avoid the splashback, Stephen, and I, the runt of the litter, half John's size (an advantage which, as I pointed out at the time, guaranteed my failure to place). John would have allowed me a handicap based on my height, but Stephen pointed out, perfectly justly, that I could have been given a two-foot advantage and I'd still never match the epic force generated by their bladders in full flow.

Perhaps he was hoping to provide a new topic for our flagging conversation? Who knows what was on his mind. He looked up, around the room, his eyes clouded and uncertain.

And this certainly was something to talk about. Almost unprecedented. It's not every day your older brother whips out his penis in mixed company.

There was a moment, a fractured second of silence. Shirley's hand went up to her mouth, but she was too late to hide the smile. She managed to hold back the laughter. Shirley always says what's on her mind. I don't know if this is a gift of her tumour. Her filter seems to have been removed with her brain tumour, which allows her to speak her mind freely.

"He's done this before," she said. "Last week. Bold as anything." She'd left her friend to keep John company while she went to the loo. John stood and stripped.

Sally glanced over to me. "Do you think he needs the loo?"

I doubted it, but being the only male in the room it was clearly my job to find out. I walked to the bedside. Shirley and her friend stepped back to let me pass.

"Do you want the loo?" I stooped to help him up, pulled his hand away from his crotch, and helped him stand, shuffled him toward the foot of the bed. There was a small ensuite bathroom at its foot. I shuffled him to the edge of the bowl, helped him with his boxers, and waited.

It was unexpected, of course. That goes without saying. I can remember a time when I still couldn't be trusted to visit the toilet by myself, a time when I had to stand on tiptoe to dangle my winkle over the cold rim of the porcelain, when it was John taking me to the toilet. Watching over me to make sure my aim was true. Nobody ever imagines this turning of tables. And of course I was uncomfortable with it. Slightly repulsed. I recognized, even as I stood there and watched and waited for the stream to begin, all that had been lost in this moment. But I dutifully waited too. Because we must, mustn't we? Tend to our loved ones. Watch their dignities stripped away from them, shred by shred. Take those steps down with them, backing down, or backing up toward total helplessness.

Nothing. Not even a couple of drops. He didn't want the loo then. I took him back to the bed, and he drifted away, half awake, half asleep, in his own little world, actually in hospital robe and boxers, on the bed. Half an hour later, he stirred again, and pointed to me at the foot of the bed. It was as if he wanted to tell me something, but couldn't find the words, forgot what he meant to say, or simply didn't have the strength. Sally tried to get him to write it down, or point to the alphabet to spell it out. I never did find out what he was trying to tell me, through the fog and confusion.

We left that evening, with a promise to return the next day.

Back at the hotel, Natalie and I discussed John's "condition," a neutered word that masks the sheer bloody horror that lies just beneath its surface. He could barely speak, had spent most of the time we were with him asleep, and when he was conscious seemed confused and withdrawn. Natalie called Larry, still at that point her boss at the Latner Centre. She described John's condition. He told her, "He doesn't have long now, from the sound of it." Confusion and disorientation are common signs that the patient is closing in on death. She told him John was still being fed by tube. "Why?" he asked. It was surely time to stop.

It goes against all instinct. Or is it instinct? Perhaps not. One of the many books I read about death during Larry's illness told the story of warriors who take themselves off to die when they feel their strength waning. So maybe our instincts are culturally determined after all. To keep our loved ones alive at any cost. To exercise all of our resources and technologies in the service of prolonging their life. To do any less is to let them down when they are at their most vulnerable. They can't fight for themselves any longer, so we must fight for them.*

It's a subject that is often misunderstood, by loved ones and relatives, but also by people who we might expect to know better: politicians and activists. They worry we starve the dying. Kill them, in fact, by withholding food. It became a component of the physician-assisted death debate in Canada. But it's a misunderstanding that stems from ignorance. An ignorance of the process of dying.

We've lost touch with death, because we never see it anymore. We've sanitized it, tidied it away out of our sight. No one dies at home anymore.

* In this we're encouraged by physicians who want to continue to actively treat patients who are patently dying. Sherwin Nuland explained the dynamic that drives physicians to continue to treat the dying in his honest account of dying and death, *How We Die.*

CHAPTER 12

Treatment

Larry and I were due to meet again on Friday (May 31), a week after our last meeting. I turned up at 9:30, as usual, but there was no answer. I pulled out my phone and called Larry's number. I could hear the phone ring inside the condo, but after a few rings it went to voicemail. Natalie works from home most Fridays, so I called her. Perhaps Larry had called to cancel after I left? No, she said. There had been no call.

My first thought was there had been some kind of medical emergency, and Faye and Larry were at a downtown hospital. But the imagination, especially when it has nothing else to do, is adept at spinning far more macabre scenarios, and it didn't take long for my heart rate to rise, and a light film of sweat to spread up my back, across my forehead and front lip. I called Larry's number again. Still no answer. Then Natalie. Still no news.

I waited in the hallway for ten or fifteen minutes, and aroused the suspicions of various diminutive, fine-boned, and frail old ladies. Finally, I left.

Fifteen minutes after I arrived back at home Faye called. Larry had been asleep in the condo and neither my raps on the door nor the phone had roused him from his slumber. It wasn't the chemo — he wasn't due to start that up again until the following week. He was just tired all the time. He had dropped off. I said I'd be happy to make the journey back to see Larry, but Faye thought it best to rearrange. Which we did, for the Friday of the following week.

In the meantime Larry's birthday, his sixty-seventh, was fast approaching. Natalie and I grappled with an unforeseen dilemma. This would be his last. Should we pretend we hadn't noticed, or tackle the issue head on? We planned on sending him an e-card, because our next meeting was two days after the big day. We'd subscribed to one of the many e-card sites because, with family scattered all over the globe, I'm never organized enough to remember to get cards into the post on time. I scrolled through the options, opening animation after animation. There was one with an old woman tending her garden. When the grim reaper confronted her she dispatched him, ninja style. The card's sign off message was: "Congratulations on beating death for another year." I played it for Natalie. "What do you think?"

"I don't know. Might be a little too close to the mark."

Larry was happy to discuss his death and he had a well-developed sense of humour. There was every chance he'd have found it funny. But there was a slim chance he might not. And there was Faye to consider. When I looked at it from Faye's perspective I could see it was far from funny. Could only be funny if it were true, and in Larry's case it wasn't. But it seemed both cowardly and at odds with the way Larry approached his death to avoid the issue completely. So we settled for a card that made a tangential reference to it — a box of eggs, and their collective realization that they're all going to die when their friend is removed from the box to make the mixture for the birthday cake.

When we met that Friday (June 7) we'd just started to chat when Larry confronted the dilemma that had almost paralyzed us when we picked out a card for him.

"Nothing major happened this week, I was just busy. It was my birthday on Wednesday. We went out in the evening to celebrate. It was another one of those bittersweet tears moments where you realize this is the last.... Everybody says happy birthday and many more of them, and you suddenly realize the many will definitely not translate. So I did a little piece in my journal on tears, because there were tears of grief and the bittersweet tears too that I think are more important in helping to resolve the grief than anything else."

"Where did you go?"

"We went to Scaramouche," a high-end restaurant at St. Clair West and Avenue Road in Toronto. "The kids were there. The girls are growing up amazingly quickly. My granddaughter was worried about the cost of the food. She looked at the menu and said 'Can I really order this? Look at the price. It's $28, you know.' No, I told her, you can actually order that."

It was hard to believe this was the man who a month previously was laid so low by jaundice that people worried he wouldn't see out the end of May. There were times then when it looked as if Larry might not make it to this milestone.

I was tempted to compare this birthday celebration with John's sixty-third birthday three years previous. Certainly, John's condition was significantly worse than Larry's. It simply would not have been possible for him to have eaten out at a restaurant, any restaurant, let alone a high-end one. And then there was the socioeconomic distance between the two men to take into account. John was comfortable in a pub. I couldn't imagine he'd have been comfortable in a silver-service restaurant. Not that he wouldn't have known what cutlery to use. It just wasn't his world. But, when you strip it down, it wasn't the calibre of the restaurant that made Larry's birthday special to him. It was the fact that he spent it surrounded by his family: his wife, his children, and his grandchildren. It was sitting together around a table, sharing food and stories. Was this not available to John too? Not really. In a long-term care home, peopled by patients in various stages of dementia, some with mental-health problems, it wouldn't have been possible to gather together around a meal and share the company of the family. Added to this, his Oldham family had to take three buses to the home, which was a significant deterrent to visiting. It didn't stop them coming, but it made their visits less frequent.

Larry turned the conversation to his grandchildren. He was clearly worried about them. He'd called on the help of the counsellors at the Latner Centre's Children's Grief Program, the Max and Beatrice Wolfe Children's Centre (which has since become Dr. Jay's Place), for the resources to help them cope, because he knew better than anyone that when one of its members is dying, the entire family needs help and support — not just the patient.

Larry was back on the chemo, although he'd been skeptical about it. In fact, in our previous meeting he'd been emphatic he wasn't going back.

"It was a worry, I must admit. I was a bit anxious yesterday."

"Why put yourself through it then?"

"I guess it's a bit of guilt factor. Also, am I missing out on a chance to feel better for a little longer to get some of these things done? Perhaps give myself more time. When we were working on the memory boxes, the volunteer from Toronto Hospice asked how much time I have left, though she didn't want to. I said, I dunno, could be next week. It could be a month from now. It could be a year from now. Who knows?

"I told Malcolm [Larry's oncologist] I want to maintain control and that if it impacts my quality of life, if I'm sick for a week after the next treatment, I will not take it anymore. And he agreed. Of course, he agreed to a point. I'm on double chemotherapy now, so he said we'll cut out one of the drugs. So I said no, no, I'm going to cut it out altogether, because I'm not sure it's really doing good.

"The other reason [I decided to go back on the chemo] was my tumour markers went down, which was surprising after just two treatments. Malcolm said, 'Considering the toxicity we gave you, that's a pretty significant number.' But I made it very clear that I'm maintaining control of all this."

Larry smiled, scratched his elbow contemplatively. "He had a trainee with him, a fellow who was rather upset that I was maintaining that kind of control."

"How did he express his annoyance?"

"A lot of small things. His body language. Some of the things he said. The way he underlined 'we'll decide if you should continue on.' I said no, you're not listening. I will decide whether I'm going to continue on. But he comes from a culture where patient-centric care doesn't exist, where what the doctor says goes. So it's a bit cultural for him."

Larry recognized he posed unique challenges. "When the fellow asked, 'Do we make appointments every two weeks to see Doctor Librach?' Malcolm said no, just monthly appointments after each cycle of chemo. 'Dr. Librach keeps in contact by email,' he said, giving me one of his wry little smiles. And I do. I'll send him an email saying this last bout of chemo gave me a lot of diarrhea, just to let you know. Malcolm's very impressed. It's actually easier because he's in and out of town all the time."

I asked if the chemo has been altered at all, to take into account Larry's sensitivity to the drugs.

"Yeah, just a reduced dose for one of the drugs: the Abraxane, which is the one that I think caused most of the symptoms, although I'm not absolutely sure about that. But the other one is Gemcitabine, which is supposed to be fairly easy on people, that's what gave me all the problems last night. So I'm now classed as little-old-lady drugs or below. But they reduced the dose of Abraxane by fifty percent so it was actually only about twenty-five millilitres of drug that infused. Considering there's twenty millilitres in the tubing there wasn't much to infuse. We'll see what happens with the next session of chemo. It's weekly, so after the first one the last time I felt pretty good, but we'll see the way it goes with the next session.

"I've got two more sessions after this one and then a break. That gives you a chance for your bone marrow to recover, so I expect I will be a little more tired, but if I'm as sick as I was the last time I'm not ... it's just not worth it. Time is of the essence. Every morning I wake up and [ask myself] is it another day gone or another day more? You know, which way is it? It's that terrible uncertainty whether the glass is half full or half empty. Am I going to be okay this morning, am I going to be able to ... you know ... I was doing better [without the chemo], I wasn't having any afternoon naps and I also came out of the chemo fog. That was the other thing around the chemotherapy. If it fogs my mind like it did the last time then I will not continue on with it. My head is too important to me. I wasn't able to read, I wasn't able to concentrate, I wasn't able to ... you know, if you'd asked me a question I would lose track of it and I would lose ... couldn't find the words."

This memory provoked another for Larry. Another amusing wrinkle in the system. He leant forward, adopted his confidential tone. "But it was funny, I was in the waiting room there [at Princess Margaret Hospital] ... I filled out this survey they're doing around patient information while I waited — they're really big on patient information — and [the subject of] this survey was concerning chemo brain. But you'd never have known. They called it 'chemotherapy-induced cognitive dysfunction.' And they plan to put that up on the rack of patient information, a leaflet on chemotherapy-induced cognitive dysfunction. So if I'm a patient looking at that I'll likely not understand what cognitive dysfunction is."

"Especially if English isn't your first language, which it isn't for a lot of patients in Toronto," I said.

"Yes. Although it's going to be available in other languages eventually. But it's only available in English now."

"How could it be improved?" I asked.

"By addressing the symptoms, so people understand what it's about. It should say something like, 'Do you find it difficult to concentrate? Do you find it difficult to think?' Then it should say, 'This could be something called chemotherapy fog, or we know it as cognitive dysfunction.' And nowhere in the survey was it suggested that patients should speak to their health-care providers about it."

Larry puffed out a long breath, an indication that he was tired. It was time to bring things to a close for the day. I flipped my notebook closed. I still took notes, despite our recordings, because I didn't entirely trust the technology. Larry seemed to flip back to thoughts of his chemo, and the challenges it was posing as I tidied my equipment away. "So I took the chemo. Despite all those things I took it … I'll put up with it as long as it puts up with me."

CHAPTER 13

Home

Our phone conversation with Larry at the Oldham Travelodge helped us make sense of what we'd seen that day. Larry also prepared us for what should happen next. We returned to the long-term care home the next day, a Friday. We had longer that day, three hours or more. Our train wasn't leaving until the early afternoon.

John was unsettled, anxious. He tried to communicate with us, but we didn't understand his gestures, and he'd never quite mastered the art of making himself heard through the trach tube. Our attempts to understand descended into a macabre form of charades: John waved his hands, his arms, in increasingly large circles, and the four of us shouted random guesses. "Sounds like you're telling us to piss off," Sally said at last. It was difficult to tell if John's thin but sheepish smile was an acknowledgement of the truth, or simply amusement at how wide of the mark the answer was. I suspected it was true. We were no use to him. We couldn't help and in his more lucid moments (if there were any) he probably felt a sharp pang of embarrassment or regret. That he'd become such a burden. Was that it? He wanted to spare us?

Or was it another symptom? This restlessness, agitation, and disorientation is common at the end of life, according to Larry. In his Dying In the First Person journal, he wrote: "People become fidgety, restless, disoriented or distressed. They may feel frightened or threatened. It is also common for people near death to believe that they see things that are not there, such as animals or people who have died. They may appear confused and may not recognize familiar faces."

He had explained it to us the previous evening. Told us not to feel insulted if John didn't recognize us. Told us it's "normal." Though it was a strange new normal that was hard to accommodate. How do you respond when the person you've travelled all this way to see tells you to piss off?

If you're English, you probably do what we did. You carry on as if it hasn't happened. You deflect, do something, anything, to create a bogus busyness.

Perhaps John wanted to move? Sally asked him if he wanted to sit in the lounge with the others. He pulled a face, the face of a child who had taken its first bite of a lemon. "He stays in his room all the time," she said. "Doesn't want to socialize. The staff worry about it."

It was July, but this was Manchester, so there was a light rain falling. Maybe he wanted to sit out in the garden for a while? He didn't answer. I went to fetch a wheelchair anyway, helped him into it.

We all navigated the elevator, John in a wheelchair, me pushing him, Sally, Natalie, and Freda. I pushed him into a corner of the garden, under a large umbrella, which stood in the middle of a round metal table — the kind they put in the back gardens of country pubs in England. There were four or five of them scattered around this small square of lawn. Somebody's attempt to make the place look cheerful. A splash of colour amongst the grey tones of the sky. John was quiet. Sally and Freda struck up a conversation with one of the home's staff. She'd popped outside for a fag, sheltering under one of the other umbrellas. She had an oatiness about her, as if some of the home's colour had seeped into her. She was cheerful and chatty, happy to have work in this economy. Happy too to share stories about some of the home's nuttier inhabitants. Natalie, indignant at this breach of patient privacy, angled her head away from the woman and whispered, "Well that's inappropriate and unprofessional."

John was restless again. Perhaps he wanted to go back? As we reached the door of his room, he pulled himself out of the wheelchair. He gripped my arm and started walking, an old-man shuffle that moved him forward inches at a time, his toenails overgrown and yellow, his grip unnaturally strong, back to his bed. Sally noticed him clenching his fists. It happened more than once. She asked if he was in pain, but he shook his head, no.

A little later he gestured to me to help him out of bed. "I'll need a nurse," I said. He was fully six inches taller than me and had always been well built. He shook his head, crooked his arm to allow me to duck my head under it. I lifted expecting the sudden heft of weight to stress my core. But it was as easy as lifting Red, my one-year-old grandson. Between the tumour and the lack of nutrition, John had wasted to nothing.

I imagined he wanted the bathroom, so I steered him gently toward the room at the foot of his bed. The iron grip of his skeletal hand (where did the strength come from?) on my forearm forced me right, not left. Out into the hallway. I humoured him, responded to the pressure on my arm, which was his only means of communication. He hadn't the energy to speak, but something was driving him forward at this slow shuffle, down the home's corridors in his bare feet.

It took me a minute to realize what he wanted. He wanted me to take him home. We were making a break for it. In his boxers and hospital robe, clutching my arm with one hand and his IV pole with the other. It wouldn't have been the fastest getaway in history.

There was enough expression left in his steel-blue eyes for me to read the despair there when I told him I couldn't take him home. It was all he wanted: a need so sharp that it drove his dying body forward with unbelievable strength.

I steered him into the communal lounge instead. If long-term care facilities are God's waiting room, this was surely the front of the queue. Old dears clinging to the last frail remnants of dignity and elegance in their pale-pink cardies, with their grey curls carefully coiffed. There were many more of them than men. The men, there were a few, a very few, were ill-kempt: hair unbrushed, rose in random tufts or drooped over their ears; gappy, coffee-stained mouths, slack and wet; salt-and-pepper stubble on flabby cheeks. But it was the eyes that really haunted me. Empty. Like there was nothing behind them. Waxwork eyes, staring but not seeing. No wonder John dismissed our offer to sit with him in the lounge with that sour expression and a petulant wave of his hand. This was not company.

Back to his room. Again, it was Sally who noticed John mouthing something, not trying to huff words through the trach tube, but mouthing, inviting her to lip read. "What did he say?" I asked.

"I don't know. I think he said, 'Get me out of here.'" His eyes glazed over when she explained, again, that this was his home now. He withdrew, became unresponsive, barely present. He'd drifted away into some liminal space. He was clearly close to death.

It was time to speak up.

Natalie and I cornered one of the home's staff, a courteous and conscientious Indian man in his mid-thirties. I introduced myself as John's brother, just to clarify my right to ask the question that followed. "Why are you still feeding him? Isn't it time to stop?"

My guess is this isn't a question he hears often. We fight for our loved ones, and what most people fight for is the longest life possible. Keep them alive at all costs is, I imagine, the attitude this conscientious care-home worker most often meets. A look of surprise and (although I may have imagined this) distaste clouded his open, helpful face for a moment before the professional manner returned and he erased it.

It sounded callous, I know it did. John was dying of cancer and now we wanted to starve him to death? Just what kind of a brother was I? But Natalie and I knew what this man evidently did not. As the body prepares itself for death it shuts down. It neither needs nor uses food. We're not starving the dying to death. On the contrary, it's the body that decides it's time.

Our perspective on death was coloured by a too-intimate knowledge of palliative care. Both Natalie and I worked on an end-of-life guide for caregivers for the Latner Centre. I recalled exactly what it said: "People generally don't feel hungry or thirsty because the body's systems have slowed. The body loses its ability to use food and fluids and does not benefit from the nutrients in them."

Which is why food and drink is sometimes withdrawn toward the end. This can alarm friends and family. Larry again: "Patients with anorexia [the clinical condition of anorexia, not to be confused with anorexia nervosa, the eating disorder] do not starve to death. Because patients with advanced cancer often appear thin and wasted, especially close to death, families often feel that they have starved to death, but this is not the mechanism of their death. Trying to provide lots of food will not prolong a patient's life."

We're ill-prepared for this moment, culturally. We may not realize it, but food (the preparation of it, the consumption of it, the enjoyment of it) is probably the last true sacrament left to us in our secular world. When we have something to celebrate (a birthday, an anniversary) what do we do? We go for a meal, or prepare one to share with our loved ones. Just as Larry did to celebrate his last birthday. Just as his family celebrated the Passover. Even John's Chelsea bun craving carried with it family memories of Saturday morning visits to the local baker to purchase freshly baked buns and doughnuts. This sacramental significance of food is driven deep into every culture on the planet, and it's reflected in our language. What is a companion, but someone who we share bread with? (From the latin *com*: "together with," and *panis*: "bread"). We talk of people having "healthy appetites." Our habitual response to illness therefore is to feed our sick. To bolster and strengthen them with their favourite foods. It is not, typically, to withhold food. To starve them. Surely that will only weaken them. Why are we starving our sick to death?

It's distressing if you don't understand. Of course we want to feed someone who's ill, but when they are actively dying it won't ease their suffering and it won't extend their life. In fact it can make them feel nauseated and uncomfortable. Worse, if you feed them when they're sleepy or can't swallow properly, the food or water can get into their lungs and lead to congestion and pneumonia.

When patients can no longer eat for themselves, families often beg for nutrition to be provided through an IV drip. It's true that in certain conditions this will extend a patient's life. But the part of the patient's life we're begging our loved one's physicians to extend is the part we should all want to be swift and painless, not extended: their death. Dying is a natural process that is as much a part of life as birth. We may not recognize it as such, because we've medicalized it, shuffled it off out of sight, into hospitals, hospices, and care homes.

So yes, I was ready to fight for my brother, but what I was ready to fight for was a death with comfort and dignity, or as much comfort and dignity as possible, given the grisly cruelty of cancer.

Our cornered staff member agreed to speak to John's physician, ask if it was time to stop feeding him.

We asked about John's medications. He told us John wasn't on any pain meds, because he wasn't reporting pain. We wondered about his anxiety. Was he being given anything to reduce that? He didn't know. He would check.

I felt impotent, and because I felt impotent I was angry. Angry at the system that had failed John in almost every way possible. Failed to diagnose the cancer early enough to treat it. Failed to provide the infrastructure, care, and support to allow him to die a peaceful death with as much dignity as he might muster, surrounded by friends, family, and familiar possessions. Failed to place him correctly — in a hospice — when the hospital was done with him.

If he were in a hospice, or were being treated by a palliative-care doctor at home, his medical team would understand. They wouldn't be trying to prolong his life artificially to spare the feelings of his friends and loved ones.

This time when I said goodbye to John I was certain this would be the last time I would see him alive. He was barely there anymore. Any spark or semblance of him, the real him, had gone. I understood for the first time people's urge to put their loved one beyond this misery. Some small part of me wanted to take a pillow and place it over his face.

Put enough miles on the clock and someone close to you will end up dying a painful or distressing death. Most people of a certain age have their story: a brother, a mother, or a lover who suffered horribly and died without the right kind of care and attention.

The debate over physician-assisted death is messy, complex, and visceral precisely because it's not a debate over abstract ideas. The debate is about real lives, real people, and their stories of pain and suffering. It's a debate that can't be uncoupled from the specific details of every life and every death, something Larry knew very well. He had been impacted by two of his own cases in particular. Cases that made him rethink his position.

It's a familiar old saw in these circumstances — the one about putting them out of their misery. So I was surprised by the strong sense I had that if I'd acted on my impulse it would have been an act of mercy, would have arisen out of my love for him. Not simply because I didn't want to witness his suffering any longer. Not simply for my own convenience and peace of mind, but because there was no hope of his improvement. Only the certainty he would get steadily worse before he died.

If I'd succumbed to that temptation, I'm sure the rest of my family would have seen it that way too, but it's unlikely the law would have agreed.

Would I have felt the same way if John had received proper palliative care, either in a hospice or at home? I don't think so. His sole and constant obsession in those months was to go home. He wanted to die at home, surrounded by his family, in familiar surroundings. That he couldn't clearly added to his distress. If he'd been given palliative care it's likely his anxiety would have been treated, and the IV-delivered food and drink stopped earlier.

But this was the U.K. Everybody knows the National Health Service is falling apart thanks to neglect from successive governments, mismanagement, resource shortages, low staff morale: a cornucopia of ills. Things are different in Canada, aren't they? If my brother had been dying in a Canadian long-term care facility he would surely have had access to palliative care, wouldn't he?

Surprisingly, the answer is no. It's unlikely he would have had access to palliative-care specialists if he'd died in a Canadian long-term care facility. The doctors at the Latner Centre are not allowed to care for patients in long-term care homes, because they have their own staff physicians. Which is true. They do. Physicians who may have little or no familiarity with palliative care. Physicians who are overworked and under-resourced. Physicians who simply don't have the time to deal with the special needs of the dying.*

After our visit, Sally tried desperately to find a way to get John home. She called the Macmillan helpline, and they suggested Marie Curie nurses. She called Marie Curie to ask what the process would be, and if John would be a candidate, and was told that while they could offer twenty-four-hour care in a patient's home, it would depend on "availability." Which is another way of saying they were short staffed, and it was a more critical problem in some areas than in others. It's a familiar story, in the U.K. and in Canada. The quality of the health care you receive is dependent upon your postal code. The divide between city and country is a particularly stark one, but even within cities as large as Toronto (or Manchester) the degree of care available to you depends on where you live in the city. The notion of a public-health system that's equitable to all is a wonderful theoretical concept, but it remains strictly theoretical while such divides exist.

All hope of getting John home again before he died was extinguished with that call.

Why had it been so important to us? Primarily because we wanted to honour his final wish to die at home. But also because I knew that the setting can have a huge impact on outcomes. I thought of the palliative-care physicians I'd spoken to over the years who provided care in patients' homes. I remembered one in particular, a young woman physician, who went to visit her patient for the first time in her home and was astonished

* "While Long-Term Care Homes Have Become a Major Location of Death in Canada, Most Do Not Have Formalized Palliative Care Programs," Virtual Hospice Website. Based on The Quality Palliative Care and Long Term Care Alliance's research currently being conducted by Lakehead University.

by the artwork covering her walls. She asked her who the artist was, and the patient replied, "Why, me, dear." When you're treating a patient in their home you cannot help but see the person, as well as their condition. It impacts the physician–patient relationship, and this, in turn, influences the outcomes of care. How can it not, when we begin to see patients, at last, as people, with lives, histories, families, loves, hopes, and dreams?

Sally called the home again. She was told that John's anxiety levels had risen, so they planned to give him sedatives to calm him down. They agreed to ask the home's doctor to refer John to a hospice.

Sally then called John's social worker. "We had quite a long conversation and I was pleased she seemed to know John and his situation well. We discussed all the options I had raised with the care home. She said in her experience Marie Curie nurses only provided cover for the night shift. She said even then she'd known times when cover was expected but didn't turn up, which wouldn't work for John's situation."

Given how close John was to death she was told it was unlikely a spot would open up at a hospice in time.

She collected her thoughts into an email to my siblings and me. "John is very close to the end of his life. It doesn't seem appropriate to move him back home not only in terms of the reliability of the Marie Curie service but also whether he would get funding. We also have to bear in mind that he doesn't seem to have much time left and just the move back could further destabilize him. I have explored the alternatives but discovered what appear to be fair reasons why they wouldn't be suitable or available in John's situation. The care home is not bad, the staff are very nice."

Sally also mentioned that the social worker was going to try to get a palliative-care physician involved in John's care, a decision that enraged Larry when Natalie told him about it. "Too little, too late," was his curt summary of the situation. I'm sure John was made more comfortable by his palliative-care physician, but I don't understand why he wasn't immediately referred to palliative care when he was first diagnosed. He'd been terminal since April. Why wait three months before calling in a palliative-care doctor? Why refer him now, barely a week (as it turned out) before he died?

Larry's anger and frustration was born, in part, from his own experiences. In the early days of palliative care in Canada it was next to impossible to get some specialists to refer their patients at all, but even though the discipline has begun to lose it's "voodoo doctor" image and join the mainstream, even now it is consistently seen as something that is invoked only when the patient is on the point of death. Yet there's a large and growing body of research to show that involving palliative-care physicians earlier in the process (even when patients are still actively being treated) improves outcomes for the patient and the health-care system.* It turns out it's cheaper, and it's better for the patient. Yet, despite this evidence, palliative care is still deployed on a "when all hope fails" basis, which often means, in Larry's curt summary, "too little, too late."

In the early afternoon (Toronto time) of Wednesday, July 14, our home phone rang. I glanced at the call display as I picked it up. It was Sally.

"Hi, Sal."

She didn't respond immediately, and when she did it was in a voice that had been washed clean of every bright note, a flat, emotionless tone from the country of the mourning. She couldn't even say the words. All she could say was "it's happened."

John had died earlier that afternoon.

I didn't learn the details until long after. Five years after, when I wrote this and needed to fill in the gaps. My brother Stephen had driven up to Oldham that day to see John. His wife, Janet, texted him on the road, urged him to call her as soon as he received it. Stephen didn't see the message until he stopped for lunch at a motorway service station. He called and Janet told him that John's step-daughter Shirley had phoned after he left home. The care home had called her and asked her to get there as soon as possible. John's condition had deteriorated. They didn't think he would live more than another few hours. Stephen was still a two-hour drive from the home. He skipped lunch and got back on the road.

* Patients experience less anxiety and depression, better patient and family satisfaction, and even live significantly longer and better.

CHAPTER 14

Grief

I'm fully cognizant of the physics of the football (or, if you prefer, the soccer ball). I'd like to make that clear. I've been playing the game for over fifty years. I've a solid grasp of both the theoretical behaviour of an inflated sphere and its practical outcomes.

On the subject of dislocated joints, more specifically, fingers, I was, until the summer of Larry's illness, a little more sketchy.

So I was not attempting to step aboard the fast-moving pass my teammate made out to the left wing in my Friday night game. It's unlikely even a fully paid-up member of the cast of Cirque du Soleil would have been able to navigate such a manoeuvre successfully. I was merely trying to bring the pass under control and to move it past a defender, something I'd achieved with a favourable outcome many times. But this time instead of gently caressing the ball to slow it, I stepped on top of it. I was moving at quite a pace but, with the help of the ball, my foot accelerated, sped past the rest of my body, and took off downfield with me attached. It was like stepping on a roller skate. I was on the ground before my head caught up with the intentions of my maverick foot. The first thing to strike me as I picked myself off the pitch was that my right hand felt a little odd. As if some foreign interloper were trying to muscle in on the territory of my ring and little finger. I looked down and was interested to see that my middle finger was bent at the knuckle, at an angle of approximately ninety degrees from its customary position. There was no pain, just the oddness of a digit being where a digit didn't belong.

My first thought was that Natalie (who was standing a few yards away on the touchline) would freak out if she saw my finger misbehaving in such a manner. As I've mentioned, I was not, at the time, *au fait* with the proper protocols surrounding dislocation. It was only a joint, I reasoned. How hard could it be to pop it back? A question I should have left in the realm of the theoretical, rather than trying to explore it by experimentation. I grasped the miscreant firmly in my left hand, tugged (I vaguely recalled reading that you're supposed to do this to provide clearance for joints to pop back in place) and jerked it back in line with its partner fingers. I tried wiggling it. It didn't co-operate. It had started to expand. It was growing by the second.

I walked off the pitch toward the knot of subs and spectators on the touchline. That was when the pain, nausea, and light-headedness kicked in.

This was the first of a number of clumsy accidents I had that summer. A few weeks later, trying to swat a fruit fly away from my almost-full pint of Blanche de Chambly, I clipped the top of the glass with the back of my hand. I should have let the glass fall, but instead tried to catch it. It shattered in my hand, spilling most of the pint down Natalie's dress and neatly slicing a three-stitch incision in the little finger of my left hand. The middle finger of my right was still in a splint. We were both surprised the emergency doc at St. Michael's wasn't more interested in exploring questions of domestic abuse, given that we'd clearly been bathing in beer and mutilating my hands.

It was most unlike me. I've never been accident prone, but in the summer of 2013 the world presented itself to me as an almost infinitely stocked repository of potential pratfalls and minor collisions. I started to wonder if it had anything to do with Larry and his condition, although it seemed unlikely. Why would Larry's illness make me suddenly clumsier? So I suppose I was more than usually alert to the subject when I stumbled upon a passage in Heather Robertson's book on death, *Meeting Death: In Hospital, Hospice and at Home*. "I remember," Robertson wrote, "that for more than a year after my mother's death, my father would fall and injure himself, something he had never done before and stopped doing later."

Her father's clumsiness occurred after her mother's death, not during her illness. But it struck me that if this was an artifact of grief it wouldn't necessarily only manifest itself *after* death. Grief can as easily hit us even while our loved ones are still living. Grief attaches itself to dying, as well as to death.

Further probing revealed that it's not just clumsiness. After her husband's sudden death from a heart attack, Joan Didion walked a similar path to that of Heather Robertson's father. In her memoir of the year following his death, *The Year of Magical Thinking*, Didion quotes the findings of a compilation of research from the U.S.'s Institute of Medicine: "Research to date has shown that, like many other stressors, grief frequently leads to changes in the endocrine, immune, autonomic nervous and cardiovascular systems; all of these are fundamentally influenced by brain function and neurotransmitters."

Knowing that grief profoundly influences the functioning of our minds and bodies may not help us very much of course. But it may help (as it helped Joan Didion) alleviate the feeling of dismay that you can no longer even stand up straight anymore.

Larry barely raised an eyebrow at my splinted finger when we met for our next meeting, the following Wednesday. After seven full days of dull gloomy weather, Toronto shone, newly minted by the sun, that morning. I didn't need a coat, which was a welcome change. Even the light breeze was welcome. Larry, who greeted me in the lounge when I arrived, was dressed for the warmer weather: olive-green shorts and a linen collarless shirt, calf-length socks. But there was something missing in his voice, an absence of its usual bright tone.

He'd started chemo again the previous week, on June 6, so he was due for another session the next day in this, his second round of chemo. We were at the point where we both realized there was no time for the subtle minuet around the subject. It was time to be direct. To ask the hard questions. So I asked him what was bothering him.

"I'm just a little more emotionally down this week," he said. "I just find that … I'd hoped that the chemotherapy would … uh … not drag me down. And I see it dragging me down after one treatment at half dose and I don't like what I feel."

The little-old-lady chemo shouldn't have done this to him. His oncologist thought it unlikely he'd suffer any of the grisly side effects normally associated with chemo. He suffered all of them. He only underwent the treatment to help him manage his symptoms, not to save his life. But it didn't seem to help him.

"So I'm waiting for my blood tests to see whether my hemoglobin has gone down, because if it has gone down significantly then I've got a real problem. They have a real problem. But I've been down. I just haven't felt well. We had friends over for dinner last night, which was fine, they left at about 7:30 and I was totally exhausted, as I usually am at 7:30."

He was also worried about a dinner date that night. It played on his mind. "We are supposed to go out and see some friends who are just around the corner, so we decided we would go to their place for dinner just to get me out. I haven't been out of the apartment now since Sunday, so I feel a little bit claustrophobic. On the other hand, I feel weaker and I don't know how much I can do out there. But I'm not in more pain. I've had nausea for two mornings in a row connected with my constipation. I've had to take Gravol, so if I take a Gravol it makes me sleep. It's a great sleeping tablet for me. I really don't feel as well as I did last week at this time, but that was before the chemo. I don't want to blame it all on the chemo, but it looks like I'm going to have to make some decisions."

He mentioned his hemoglobin levels were low. He forgot sometimes that I'm not a doctor. I know hemoglobin is the protein in red blood cells that carries oxygen through the body, so it's obviously nice to have plenty of it, but I didn't understand the significance of low hemoglobin levels. What did it mean?

"It means my bone marrow is being suppressed. It means I can't take the chemo, at least in the doses they've given me. So that's the problem. And I don't want to bounce way down, which leaves me open to serious risk because it's not only that your hemoglobin's down, but your white counts, your platelets ..."

He remembered this time to explain the consequences of these conditions. The low white count put him at high risk from any infection, even a cold, because he wouldn't have the resources to fight it. Because that's what the white blood cells do. The low platelet count meant his blood would have trouble clotting, so he was at high risk of bleeding.

"And I have a tumour that is known to cause bleeding. So you know, what do I want to do with that? What are the risks? That's something I look at.... Before they even put the first bag of chemo up, I ask to see my blood results and see what it shows, because if it's significantly down I won't take the chemo. Not without speaking to my oncologist. If it's significantly down, which it wasn't with the first chemo the last time, then it just means my bone marrow reserves are very limited. That's been weighing on my mind."

"So that brings up that question of control," I said. We'd discussed it earlier, but this seemed a perfect example of Larry's ability to keep a measure of control over his treatment. "People will say, well that's okay for Larry Librach to decide he doesn't want the chemo, he's a doctor, he's a very eminent man, of course his doctors will accede to him, but what about me? I don't have any medical degrees ... how do I take control of the situation?"

"It's true. The message is always listen to your doctor. But at this stage you're not dealing with a cold, you're not dealing with a mild illness, you're dealing with your death, or impending death from a disease that is eventually going to kill you. People do have the power to say stop, you know? They just don't realize it and the settings that they are in may not give them the opportunity." By settings Larry meant the venue: hospital, hospice, care home, or home. "So you're right, because of the field I'm in I find I can say no. Because I have the experience, I can say, 'Hey, look, what am I going to do with an extra month of life if I can't think?' And the other thing that has happened over the past week is the chemo fog's returned ... so you may find that I lose track of questions and words because that's started to set in too."

"And you've already said you're not prepared to —"

"Not prepared to have it as bad as it was the last time, yeah. But people do have the power."

There it was, Larry's chemo fog. He'd always had the kind of butterfly mind that would jump from topic to topic, but he'd typically finish a thought before starting a new one. So we settled back on the petals of the last subject, exercising control over your care and treatment. I'd been thinking about this since our last discussion, and I had a theory to run past him: that the institution, and its rigid control of and insistence on its rules and protocols, browbeats patients. Is, in fact, explicitly designed to send a not-so-subtle message: you (the patient) have no power or will outside of that small latitude we may deign to grant you. It's what Larry meant when he talked about "settings." If the setting is the hospital, for example, it's much harder for patients to advocate for themselves.

He nodded. "They [patients] do seem to be powerless to act, they seem … as soon as they put those wristbands on … it suddenly jails them."

"It may sound trivial," I said. "Silly even. But they make patients gown up, even when it seems utterly unnecessary. Why? Because it puts the patient at a disadvantage. Street clothes help us project ourselves, in some small way help us define ourselves, to ourselves and to others. They reflect our character. The way we dress, the way we hold ourselves, says something about who we are. So if you strip that away and dress everyone in the same dowdy, threadbare hospital robe, you've redefined the power structures in the relationship. You're in charge. It's much harder to be dignified and self-assertive in flimsy old cotton rag, with your bottom hanging out the back."

Larry nodded as I made my point. "It is demoralizing for patients. The Holocaust survivors used to hate the wristbands we put on because it reduced them to a number and that was the way the Nazis dehumanized them. Actually, when you are in the hospital you are reduced to a number. What's your medical records number? How the hell do I know my medical records number? It's on my wristband. But that's right, the things we do, I mean we put people in the hospital rooms that don't have private washrooms. We have loud noises outside. We don't respect the hospital quiet rules. We leave them out in cold corridors with little air to breathe. There's been lots written about hospitals and the demoralizing effect they have. If you're lying there with a terminal illness, you may not care or you may care a lot. For me, I do care a lot about things. For the first few days I was in hospital I didn't bring any pajamas or anything with me, so I was in hospital gowns, freezing to death one minute, sweating the next. I was in hospital gowns and they were bothering me. Oh it was awful."

"They're not the most comfortable garments are they?"

"And these days the hospitals try to preserve laundry so they don't like giving you more than one sheet a day or more than one gown. That's the way things are. It doesn't make a difference whether you're a palliative patient or any other kind of patient. Although some hospitals in the U.S. have really progressed; they give you gowns that actually feel like a gown. They actually wrap around the front." A small concession perhaps, but a humane one.

I was attending the Canadian Authors' Association's conference in Orillia that weekend, but Natalie kept me up to date with Larry's condition. Her office was a step across the road from PMH, where Larry took his chemo, and old friends from the Latner Centre were always dropping in on him when he was there, so she knew before me that the following day he was at Princess Margaret. She messaged me on my phone as soon as she heard.

His numbers must not have been as bad as he suspected they might be. But I'll admit to having a twinge of doubt at the news, and I'm not afraid to admit it was mixed with a little fear for him. The chemo had brought him down with a crash before. I feared it might happen again.

CHAPTER 15

The War on Cancer

One of the many hazards faced by patients undergoing chemo is neutropenia, a shortage of neutrophils, the white blood cells responsible for fighting the body's infections. Chemo tends to knock out neutrophils, so it's routine to check a patient's white-cell count before every cycle of chemo. If the white count is too low, the chemo will be cancelled.

It happened to Larry in late June. While they checked his white count, they administered Decadron, a steroid that is supposed to counterbalance many of the worst effects of the chemo, such as nausea and tiredness. His white count was too low, so the chemo was cancelled.

But Decadron has an unfortunate side effect: it can make sensitive patients tweaky and restless. Larry was hypersensitive to the chemo. So when I visited him the next day he seemed super-caffeinated, talking at an almost manic pace. "I was on a tear yesterday. I went up to Yorkdale and I walked all over the mall. I think I exhausted myself.

"I knew that my counts were way down this week." He offered me his palms, swivelled his wrists to demonstrate how white they were, how low his hemoglobin levels must have dropped.

It had been nine days since our previous meeting. Whenever there was a long gap between our meetings the changes he'd been going through were always more noticeable. Today his hair loss was much more evident. It was already thinning, even in May, but now his scalp was shining through the sparse fuzz that chemo had left to him. And he was losing weight in his face. It had an odd effect, making his head seem smaller, more wizened.

Was the chemo still working? I asked. Had they run the numbers on his tumour markers lately?

"They only do those once a month, so they won't be done until the first week of July. We'll see. They haven't done a CT scan either. I'm in two minds about doing a CT scan. It's either going to be good news, bad news, or no news, and none of those really help me, because you don't know what's going on. In fact, if it's more bad news, it's just … it will send my mind spinning, and I don't need that."

Why submit to the tests then, if there's nothing to be gained from taking them? Because he was right, given his prognosis, what was to be gained by simply measuring the steady march of his disease?

"My family wants the results. With patients you see this all the time. We over-investigate people, sometimes because they want to know, but to be honest with you, when you look at results, unless there's been a huge remission, like a fifty percent decrease in the tumour size … if there's a slight increase or slight decrease or no change it means nothing to the prognosis. It doesn't really tell you anything. And even in remission it doesn't tell you that the remission is going to last, or what does that mean? Or what if you get new metastases?"

It was that duplicitous monster again: hope. The hope there would be a miracle, that the tumour might have retreated, that Larry might beat the odds, might be one of the two people in a hundred who survive this cancer. It happens. Why not? Larry himself had doggedly refused to hope for this, had insisted on rationality over faith, on reason over magical thinking, on the implacable nature of this particular cancer. But he was sympathetic to this weakness in others.

I asked him how he was tolerating the chemo, apart from the neutropenia.

"Over the week I wasn't too bad. I was surprised. Though I have to push myself to avoid napping in the afternoon, unless I absolutely have to. And I have to push myself to keep doing the things I'm setting out to do. I think we accomplished a fair a bit last week. I didn't get out much, because the weather was funny."

Even though Toronto had a relatively wet summer in 2013, the week had been hot and humid.

"But there are things to do here, and visitors have picked up again. It's fun having visitors. I don't mind that. I've been on the phone some more with people, and some new people have reached out to me, which has been interesting."

Larry had mentioned, back in May, that some of the younger physicians at the Latner Centre struggled with how to deal with his cancer, or more particularly with the fact that he was dying. They didn't know what to say. He wrote an entry in his journal about it:

> *Considering that many of my friends are palliative-care professionals and spend their working lives talking to dying patients, I find it interesting that even they have difficulty expressing their words to me.*
>
> *The thing that is most comforting is the fact that they are in contact whether it is by email, telephone, Skype, or written letters. In my periods when I am very afraid of my impending death, re-reading those emails and other contacts soothes my soul. It is my sense of the "afterlife."*

It comforted him that the younger staff at the Latner Centre were "finally losing their fear of [him]." Other physicians at the Centre had been in touch too. They were fascinated to know how Larry, knowing what he knew, managed to keep enough to himself so he didn't overburden his family, and yet still got the support he needed from them. I asked him how he walked that line.

"I've been lucky. Faye and I have our daily forever hug and cry, but we have other times when we talk about it and times when I have tears that I keep to myself. And then there are times when I have tears that just flow."

He mentioned one colleague, Anne Langlois, who had been particularly interested in how he maintained this balance. She had emailed him often in the previous few weeks. "It's interesting, because it truly is a balance. People look at cancer as fighting 'the battle.'" He drew the quote marks in the air with his forefingers. This was something we'd discussed before, so I knew exactly what he meant. The language that enfolds cancer and cancer patients is the language of warfare. People talk of "fighting" cancer, or "winning" or "losing" their "battle" against it. In his book *The*

Emperor of All Maladies, Siddhartha Mukherjee argued that this rhetoric of the "war on cancer" came out of the U.S. and its Nixon-era push to find a cure for cancer.

It's a rhetoric Larry believed damages patients and physicians alike. "I think it sets you up for defeat right away, because it's really not a battle. It's a health challenge. You work with it, like diabetes or heart disease." The problem with the warfare rhetoric is that if you lose your battle "you feel like you're a loser, and the only losers in this are the patient and family. If it's a health challenge you can work through it and at least you have the idea you have done something. So Anne and I have been having a great conversation in email and I hope she'll follow it up with a visit because not a lot of my colleagues have been able to speak like that. Albert Kirshen does, David Kendal does, Russell does, and so does Sandy, but they are older physicians with more experience. I think that makes a difference to their approach and their ability to talk about things."

"Do you think perhaps the younger physicians are intimidated by your reputation?"

"I think so. I had an email from Ramona [Mahtani] this morning in which she said something like that." Ramona was one of the last physicians Larry appointed when he was director of the Latner Centre. They worked together for a year before he retired in 2011. "She said she'd admired me from afar, that I've been a leader and a mentor to her. [So it may well be that] they are afraid to approach me. And when they do approach me, I seem to have the answers and they're thinking whoa, well they don't have the answers so there's something wrong. I think they just don't have enough experience under their belt. Part of it is that they put me on a pedestal, which is what medicine has done far too much. You know, you're the great god Librach up there, and those things ... they inhibit people. I've always tried to push myself down. I don't believe in hierarchies. But I grew up with professors who imposed a definite hierarchy — that's the British system. So I think it's a matter of [them gaining] the confidence that I don't bite. Sometimes when I have worked with younger physicians I've overcompensated and provided them with the answer rather than have them work their way through it. Most of the time I've been right about what has to be done, but if I've been wrong they haven't told me either."

That week the news had been dominated by Quebec's end-of-life bill (Bill 52, which passed into law in June 2014). Bill 52 has long since been overtaken by other events, because in February 2015 Canada's Supreme Court overturned a previous ruling that outlawed physician-assisted death in Canada. The Court's ruling had a one-year time fuse attached to it. It did not come into effect until February 2016. But Quebec's Bill 52, in some sense, prepared the way. It made physician-assisted death legal in Quebec over eighteen months before the Supreme Court decision would make it legal across Canada. Larry didn't live to see the Supreme Court's decision. That was still over eighteen months in the future. However, he'd provided evidence to the justices who delivered that ruling.

Dr. Kerry Bowman, Mount Sinai's clinical bioethicist, had been interviewed about the bill and its implications on *CTV News* that morning. I asked Larry what he thought about the bill, and especially what he thought about its implications for palliative care.

"They are going to do it and it's going to cause all sorts of distress."

"Kerry Bowman made a good point," I said. "He said we should be thinking a bit more about palliative care, rather than physician-assisted death. That's where he said the emphasis should be placed."

"Well, yeah, he's right. Ten years ago if you had asked if I were in favour, I would have said no way. But I've watched too many people suffer too much. Even when people are receiving the best of palliative care, and I've had patients like this — actually," Larry cracked one of his smiles, "I provided the care, so it was obviously excellent — there is a certain amount of psychological and physiological and physical suffering that people go through.

"One case that really started me thinking differently was a man in his fifties who developed pancreatic cancer. He was a healthy man. Used to jog ten kilometres every day. He owned a fabulous company and was the nicest guy. He was referred to me. He lived outside our normal area, but I took the case as a favour to friends. And I met this guy, he was a wonderful guy, but they sent him home from hospital. He had a complete bowel obstruction. He couldn't put anything in without vomiting it up. He lived in this gorgeous house north of Steeles, and when I walked through the door the first thing he asked me was, 'Are you going to help me die?' I couldn't quite gather what he was talking about. We talked and we hit it off very well … but after a couple of weeks he said, 'Lookit, I've done everything you said I should do …' and he had. He'd spoken to his two daughters, and he'd spoken to his wife about what he wanted, and he'd done all the background legal stuff. He'd gone into work and had taken each one of his forty-seven employees and sat down with each one of them over a period of two weeks and said how important they had been to the business … from the guy in the stock room or the mailroom to his VPs … and how he wouldn't be involved anymore. His wife was going to be taking over the company. Everything was set and they shouldn't worry about their jobs. And he said to me, what is there waiting for me? Now, unlike me — I don't have complete bowel obstruction — we knew that he was going to perforate his bowel and die of peritonitis. [There was a slim possibility] he was just going to go on and die a nice, gentle death. But it was more likely he was going to die of peritonitis. So I talked to him about this and said it's a possibility. I told him we'd continue his terminal sedation and make sure that he'd be unconscious during this period of time, and that his pain control would be good. So he said to me, 'Well, how do you know when this is going to happen?' I said when it happens, it will happen pretty suddenly, and we'll have all the stuff here. He says, 'How can you guarantee that everything will work by the time it has to work, and that I won't suffer too much? It means I just have to lie here in bed and I'm worried about my family and I'm worried about me and it's just dragging on. Why can't you help me die?' I said we'll put you in continuous palliative sedation and you will die during that and we won't give you any food or fluids." Palliative sedation (also known as terminal sedation) is a last-gasp measure that's given to the imminently dying. It's used on patients with intractable pain or other stubborn or unmanageable symptoms like shortness of breath. Simply put, the patient is put into a deep sleep, usually with a subcutaneous sedative (or sometimes with an intravenous drip). It's a sleep from which they will not wake. But that wasn't enough for Larry's pancreatic cancer patient. "He said, 'Can you help me die before that?' And every time I walked into the house — I did weekly home visits for the next five weeks — I said look, we've got everything here, but I can't help you die. And sure enough one weekend he perforated his bowel. By the time the on-call physician got up there he was in absolute agony. There's nothing worse than having acid and bowel contents in your peritoneum. I know,

I had peritonitis during my jaundice incident. And before she could get enough medication into him, he died in agony.

"After this, I used to see his wife occasionally and she would just turn her back on me. So that was the thing that said to me, well, maybe I was being too rigid.

"I had another patient, and the same thing. He was dying of bowel cancer, which had metastasized to his lungs. And he was worried because he had watched his father suffocate to death with lung cancer. And I said no, that's not going to happen to him, and of course it did happen to him. I would go to visit, but I couldn't help this guy. I spent hours at his home as he died, watching him suffocate. I couldn't control it. And so I said, am I being so rigid that I have to think that my views have to supersede somebody else's?" In Larry's view his patient had done everything he'd asked of him. He'd done everything right. But he was facing death by torture. How could it be the right ethical choice to force him to suffer through that, having used medical science to keep him alive as long as he had?

"So when I was president of CHPCA we started a task force on assisted dying," Larry said. The euthanasia and assisted-suicide task group's job was to monitor developments and come up with policy recommendations. "I said, look, everybody in palliative care will say we can't get involved. But we are going to get involved because who within the medical establishment knows better about dying than we do? But I firmly believe you need a good palliative-care system before you allow assisted death. Otherwise people will be forced into it and they don't have to be."

Which raises the critical question: now that we've made assisted death legal, what's to stop the greedy and the unscrupulous from abusing it? It's much more expensive to provide palliative care for six months, a year, two years, so why not just shuffle the sick and the dying off the conveyor belt? Decrease the load on the health-care system, decrease the need for hospice and hospital beds. Save ourselves the trouble and expense of dealing with the terminally ill by anticipating nature, or hurrying it along. Of course, that's a caricature of a certain strand of the argument, but the worry over potential abuse is real.

Larry didn't accept this argument.

"The experiences in Oregon and Washington have shown that out of the hundred people who get approval for this — and you have to meet certain criteria — only five percent ever access it. It's a very good system. They aren't going after the elderly and they're not going after the disabled. There is always the slippery slope argument that we'll descend into a Nazi hell. I think that speaks of lack of confidence that our society can protect. We do such a good job in protecting people. So I think it's a spurious argument."

But Larry recognized it would be controversial in the world of palliative care. "It's a problem. Lots of people in palliative care are very religious. Less so now, but it was started by people with heavy religious backgrounds. Dame Cicely Saunders at St. Christopher's Hospice, for example. To be honest with you, I got tired of working with those people because they couldn't accept anything."

I wasn't sure what Larry meant. He reminded me that palliative care is fraught with ethical dilemmas. For example, what if a pregnant woman has cancer and the chemo will kill her unborn child? Do you try to save her or her child? His religious colleagues and their decisions were being led by religious, rather than medical, considerations. "It was all God," Larry said. "I said seventy-five percent of the population is secular, so start thinking beyond God. To this day there is one brilliant palliative-care physician who used to be a friend of mine who won't talk to me because I opened up the discussion on physician-assisted death.

"Ultimately, all the CHPCA task force did was look at what the issues were and said very clearly it's not a role of palliative care to be forced to do assisted-death. But the thing that we have to worry about is to make sure that there's a system out there that will protect those that are dying. So in Oregon, you have to be referred for palliative care before you can consider physician-assisted death. You don't have to accept it, but you have to be assessed and you have to know what it's all about and you have to be aware of that. And almost all of the people who are accepted for assisted-suicide are in a hospice program."

It's important to remember that in the U.S. palliative care is often referred to as hospice care. People in hospice programs aren't necessarily in a hospice. They may be receiving treatment at home, or in nursing homes or long-term care facilities. A similar subtle, but important, semantic distinction needs to be made between physician-assisted death and euthanasia. The most common distinction between the two terms focuses on who administers the medication. Physicians administer the medication in euthanasia. In physician-assisted death the physician's role is that of a facilitator. He or she will weigh the merits of the case, and agree to write the prescription (or deny the request), but the medication is administered by the patient or a volunteer.

"In Oregon the physician writes the prescription and then he is not supposed to have anything more to do with the process. It's done by volunteers," Larry told me. "The patient has to be able to administer the medication herself. They choose the time and the place. It's almost always done in the patient's home. A volunteer can mix it up. It's a hundred capsules of barbiturates and it tastes terrible, but you are dead in ten minutes. There have only been a couple of cases in all the times they've had it done where somebody has survived. You just never know people's way of handling drugs. Barbiturates are the most reliable way of doing things. Other medications aren't half as good.

"In Switzerland the patients have to be competent. The volunteer makes up the medication, and attaches it in an IV. The patient is the one that presses the button that injects the medication. It's often a family member that helps press the button as well. They are dead in minutes. In Switzerland they often do it in rented apartments until people in the neighbourhood find out about it. It's become a problem, suicide tourism, people are going there from Canada ... there was a case in the newspapers recently ... a woman went and arranged for assisted death because she couldn't get the help here in Canada. Oregon doesn't allow that ... you need to be a resident. In Washington, the same. Montana, interestingly enough, has no legislation governing it, but their Supreme Court has said that it's legal. They have developed guidelines, but they have no legislation. There are a couple of other states looking at it.

"There is no doubt that a lot of physicians already feel like they have assisted people's death by withholding and withdrawing treatment, but that's legal and ethically sound. It's on a whole spectrum of things. It's not just a simple sort of yeah, we'll do it or not do it ... even terminal sedation can be seen ... because you are withdrawing food and fluid. People don't last a long time. You're giving it in the last two weeks of life and people are going to die, and it takes some time to die anyways, but it is not the instantaneous thing you get with the usual assisted death protocol.

"Assisted death is the next big thing. It's interesting that the Quebec government is saying it's not a legal issue because they can't change the law. The law is national ... it's federal. They are saying it's a health-care issue. I think the government will try to ... I think they have to take it to federal court first of all ... to say that it's federal jurisdiction. In the meantime in Quebec the palliative-care society says it's totally against it. I know other people in Quebec who disagree. They say, well, you know, if it came in it would be good for palliative care."

And it will, Larry said. Bill 52 is not a physician-assisted death charter. It deals with all aspects of end-of-life care, and mandates that patients should have access to palliative care. "So it means the Quebec government, because they are further behind than almost every province in palliative care, will now have to provide it. So I think it's good for the feds. There are already the two cases before the Supreme Court. I gave an affidavit on one of them, which has been widely quoted. It was really around the issues, saying that people can get the best of palliative care and there still would be a few people for whom that's not enough. Why do we, as a society, force them to be in pain? Because there are people with intractable pain. They say they can't stand it anymore. They want relief of pain and they're not depressed. I think we are going to, within the next ten years, see a system of assisted death that will be protective."

Larry believed the general public is more sanguine about our abilities to put checks and balances in place, and provide safeguards against abuse. A view that was borne out by a number of public polls on the topic. "You're finding a lot of support [for physician-assisted death] within the Canadian public. But although people say that they would access it, when you are there, it's very different."

For Larry the increasingly entrenched pro-life and pro-choice positions both failed to accommodate the subtle nuances of the debate. For them the choice is binary — to kill or not to kill — but Larry believed it's a spectrum of choices that will constantly move and evolve as technological change puts new, and tough, ethical choices into the hands of our physicians. In other centuries Larry's lung-cancer patient would have died long before his cancer-riddled lungs suffocated him. Medical science kept him alive long enough for him to die an agonizing death by drowning in his own fluids.

My own perspective was shaped by watching John suffer during the final stages of his illness. The almost instinctive response of alleviating suffering by terminating a life is hard to balance against medical imperatives and the current legal system. But the reality is that our ability to artificially prolong life oftentimes creates this dichotomy. And knowing when to relax our control of events and let nature take its own course is sometimes both the most compassionate and the most fitting route to the solution.

Larry understood this. He also understood that each case needs to be evaluated on its own merits. Sometimes, perhaps most of the time, the right palliative care will change the patient's mind. "It relates somewhat to the burden. If you feel that you are a total burden it might drive you to assisted death, but people see they can cope. Life has value. They can live well until they die. And sure, there's going to be some suffering, but they can cope with that. So you're weak, but you still have your head, you still have your family. So we are going to see some changes. Canada would be the first big country that has authorized it. Australia has toyed with it. One of the states in Australia legalized it and then it was thrown out federally for the same kind of argument that Quebec tried to use ... so we'll see whether that will work.

"If you walked out on the streets of Toronto and asked people you'd find there's strong support for at least giving people the opportunity. People may not understand the opportunity ... people don't understand the opportunity for palliative care."

In the event, Canada was the first big country to authorize physician-assisted death, and the ten-year timeline Larry talked about was compressed into a mere three. The Supreme Court's judgment left it to the physicians, the institutions at which they work, and provincial parliaments to work out the details of how such a system would work in practice. During the year that followed the Court's decision, they scrambled to come up with a plan. Given the patchwork quilt that is Canada's health-care system, it's likely there will be some differences in how each province legislates for it. All the agencies involved were keenly aware that they were on a countdown. As soon as the Supreme Court's one-year stop clock expired there would be patients (perhaps not many, but some) knocking on their doors, insisting upon availing themselves of the right to die.

CHAPTER 16

Chemoland

On Thursday, June 27, Larry endured the first bout of his next round of chemo. It had been almost three months since he'd been told he had only a couple of months to live. When you know your time on Earth is possibly down to a handful of days it's rational to resent anyone who wastes a day or any part of one. Larry resented the time he wasted in what he termed Chemoland.

It wasn't the first time he'd complained about the mayhem and the time he lost in the chemo suite. In early June he'd described the routine in the waiting room to me. "Everybody looks at each other to see who looks sicker this week. It seems very pleasant. It's got a couple of fake fireplaces and a big-screen television, running CP24. After five minutes you've seen all the news. One of the receptionists put on the tennis match yesterday, so that was a hit."

According to Larry the unit's cosmetic appeal masks some fundamental design flaws. "It may look nice, but it's a horror story. The chairs aren't comfortable, but then hospitals, as we found out at the Latner Centre when we moved, are restricted to certain types of chair." Natalie had once explained why. She ordered new chairs for the Centre during an office refurbishment, but her choices were limited. Patients tend to be leaky. Hygiene dictates chairs need to be wipeable, to meet certain quality standards. "Not that they hang together very well. So though the chemo unit's only two years old some of the upholstery is already cracked.

"And the waiting room is still arranged in rows: one long row after one long row, which is hard because they're so close together. If you're going down with a walker or a wheelchair, people have to squeeze in. Even with a cane that I'm using constantly now, people are still in the way."

That's if you can get a chair. On his June 27 appointment the waiting room was packed. "There wasn't a single empty chair. Which is not unusual, although it's a huge waiting room. People leaned against the wall. People sat on the floor. People sat on planters outside. And the staff's attitude was 'oh well.'"

But the thing that bothered Larry most was the wasted time. "The later you're booked the harder it is to get in on time, because everything always goes over time. I'm very parsimonious about my time. My chemotherapy was scheduled for 9:30. I arrived at 9:10." Larry habitually arrived twenty minutes before his appointment.

"You put your hospital card in the plastic box. That's the first step. Then you wait. Eventually, after another thirty minutes, they call you to get your little pager — one of those gadgets like you get in a restaurant — so they can call you when your chemo area is ready for you. The little light goes on and it buzzes. That's another sticking point. In a busy waiting room, with the registration desk way at the front and off to the side, you can't hear the names they call out, especially if you're at the back. So I get my pager and I don't get paged for thirty minutes. That's forty minutes after my scheduled time. Finally I got a seat.

"I got called to Orange 19, my personal chemo area." There are five chemo suites at Princess Margaret, and they've recently been refurbished. Two are designed for "very sick" patients according to Larry — those patients whose chemo treatment is more complex, more difficult. "The rest of us go to the orange, yellow, or purple chemo suites. They're busy places, but they're relatively pleasant, and relatively well run. The people are very good. There are a lot of people there, you've got your own primary nurse who looks after you. I've been fortunate enough to have the same nurse several times now, and she's a doll."

The chemo "rooms" are "open concept, brightly lit, with windows and multiple patients in different, closely situated areas," according to Larry's daughter, Judith. There are just two chairs, one for the patient and another for a visitor, so if someone else came to visit Larry when

Judith was there she had to leave to make room. She said it's quiet, but "not morose."

On this particular day, Larry said, "they'd tried to cram six people into an area designed for four. It was crowded with patients, visitors, equipment, nurses, and other personnel. Heaven help you if you are feeling unwell. They set up my IV and we waited, because as usual the drugs were not ready." There was a good reason for that. The meds have to be prepared. "It's an emulsion, so they have to put it in a contraption like a paint shaker to get it shaken up enough so it will stay an emulsion. That takes an hour and a quarter, and they don't make it up until you've checked in because it's expensive.

"I sat there another hour with the IV running before the drugs arrived. The infusion times are short, about thirty minutes per drug. You just sit there and let the drug go in."

Larry did his best to make use of the time. "They have a little kitchen there where you can get juices and drinks and sit with family members and friends. Almost everybody comes with somebody, which they encourage you to do because a lot of the pre-meds are such that you don't want anyone going home alone."

He took his iPod and iPad with him, but his favourite pastime was spending time with visitors. Sometimes his daughter, Judith, sometimes friends and old colleagues from the hospital. One week he had a two-hour father–daughter discussion.

"I have to say," Judith said, "it was special to be there for us, uninterrupted, relatively quiet time when there was nothing to do but sit back. It was almost like sitting in a coffee shop together: light conversation, a few jokes, and sometimes, of course, coffee."

On this particular day Larry's friend Yves Talbot came by for a few minutes: "He's a delightful friend. He's been really struck by all this.

"But it's waiting, it's always the waiting," Larry said. The preparation takes longer than it takes to infuse the drugs. It really takes no time whatsoever. It's fifteen minutes … and the washout for the Abraxane is about fifteen minutes, so it's a half hour and a half hour for the other one and you're done. The waiting is longer than the actual treatment."

"And then there's the blood. I've learned to go at off times for the blood so I just walk in and get my blood done in five minutes. If you go at the time they suggest everybody's there at the same time trying to get their blood drawn.

"I didn't get out of there until 12:45. The actual treatment time, including starting the IV and infusion, was an hour and a half, so two hours of my time was wasted. This is a normal chemo appointment.

"Surely they should be able to sort that out. We say we are patient-centred in our perspective. The system is far from patient-centred. We waste the time of patients, family, and health-care providers. The system needs an overhaul with a good review by a systems engineer, rather than the bland acceptance I saw. The attitude is, 'Well, that's just the way it is.' More patients could be handled more effectively if we truly had a sense of an efficient system and office design. Nobody in medicine — across the board — has thought in terms of human systems: performance-human-systems engineering. They've measured performance, how many minutes does it take to do things, but they haven't really looked at how everything fits together as a system, and it's obvious that cancer doesn't work as a system. It works as several disparate pieces. And the people in the system are not attuned to what's happening out there. They sit behind the desk. It's like they are sitting behind a wall in a castle with a moat outside. You take a look out there in the world the patients inhabit and you realize they're really distressed."

Larry's tone dropped an octave. "And nobody offered anything to people. Even the volunteers that go around and hand out cookies and so on. They were excessively cheerful but didn't really address the fact that people were upset and waiting. When I was finally called, the lady sat next to me had been there for three quarters of an hour longer than me. Her appointment was for nine o'clock, and she still hadn't been called. She had driven almost a hundred kilometres from Port Hope to get there on time. So she was visibly upset, but she got only shrugs from staff. She had her little pager and it still didn't ring. For her the day was already wasted. We don't have, as cancer patients, a lot of time to waste. It really demoralizes patients to see how they're treated like ... not really a number at the door. I understand why you need numbers, that may be privacy, but they yell out your numbers and it doesn't help when you have a noisy waiting room and you're at the back and you have hearing problems, when they are way at the front and the side and they don't yell out. It's just a measure of our lack of humanity in some ways in dealing with these things.

"When I was in family practice we sometimes had very busy waiting rooms. It was rare that the partner with whom I shared the practice and I were there at the same time, so if there were times when I went in and saw that 'Oh my God, there is a waiting room full of people and people are standing outside,' I'd take them and put them into the second examining room just to let them sit down. Respond to people's needs. Recognize something is a bit off and show that somebody is prepared to do a little bit to fix it. That's enough to help. Or just make an announcement to say 'Sorry folks, there's a meeting,' or 'We're having trouble getting the drugs,' or 'We're short a pharmacist,' or 'We're short a nurse,' or whatever. Just something to recognize there's a group of people hanging on your words. They just want to know what the hell is going on."

"Other than your time being wasted in chemo," I asked, "how was your week last week?"

"I had some breakthrough pain on Friday night," he said. Breakthrough pain — a spike in pain that "breaks through" the long-acting painkillers the patient is on — can be frightening, and difficult to manage. Larry's breakthrough was in his chest. He said, "I couldn't figure it out. You know, one of the things you can get with this type of cancer in particular, is blood clots. So they are always worried about blood clots in my lungs. But it didn't feel like that." Larry said he had to take some painkillers to deal with the pain. "It's very scary."

"Then, on Saturday, late afternoon, a fever struck. I started feeling very flushed, which I normally do anyways when I'm on the Decadron. I took my temperature, and I said whoa … this is strange. It was 37.9 degrees." Normal temperature for healthy adults is 37 degrees. "It was close enough to 38 to start me worrying. Within a little while it was 38, 38.1, 37.9, so I called the hospital." Princess Margaret gives all its cancer patients a binder telling them whom to call in the case of an emergency. "In my binder it says call the nursing supervisor on-call … well, I wanted to speak to the resident … why would I want to speak to the nursing supervisor? So I called her. No answer. It went to voicemail. Great. I left a message and she still hasn't called back. So that doesn't help.

"The fever came on quickly, but I was feeling okay. Maybe some chills, but I was feeling okay."

"So, you went to Emerge on Saturday?"

"Yeah, at six in the evening. As soon as you think things are nice and stable it comes around and kicks you in the backside. This fever just came out of the blue, especially because it was so close to the chemotherapy. That's not usual. I had high counts so I couldn't imagine my counts were low — they weren't."

It wasn't clear to me why he was worried about the fever when he said he was feeling okay.

"Well, because I have this stent." The stent in his bile duct that was placed there in May to fix his jaundice. "There's a condition, ascending cholangitis, that's a very dangerous infection." Indeed. It's an infection of the bile duct, classified as a medical emergency. "It would kill me quicker than the cancer. The stent's a foreign body in my body, and that attracts bacteria and weakens my defences. There isn't the same sphincter control and stuff like that.

"So we finally got out of there at 11:00–11:30 at night. It's just wasted time. I told Faye, they used to have a protocol so that cancer patients go in, and there was a protocol for neutropenic fever, or fevers in cancer patients. You did x, y, and z and called the oncology resident, who came over to see you. But when they started fiddling around with the numbers of residents in oncology they didn't have the resources anymore, so they stopped that. So we spent from six o'clock until 11:30 p.m. in Emerge. We waited three hours for a simple blood test. That was the big hold up. It was just a CBC [complete blood count], just a white count. That's all. And we waited three hours. I had just finished a section of my journal on wasted time in Chemoland because of my bad experience on Thursday with chemotherapy. It really threw me yesterday when … I was blotto, because I hadn't really slept in the night after I came back from Emerge …"

"And did they fix the fever?"

"No! It broke by itself. I had one of these hot flashes and it broke. Never did figure out what caused it. Every day counts, and to waste a significant amount of time ain't great. I used to work in the Emergency Department. I know there are delays. That was when Emergency was much less efficient. You couldn't get the blood tests online back then. But even the resident who saw me couldn't believe it took three hours to get a simple CBC. Everything else came back but the CBC. Three hours … it wasn't like they were overwhelmed in the Emergency Department."

"So how was the white count?"

"It was good. It was around seven thousand." Normal white-blood-cell count ranges from 4,500 to 10,000 white blood cells per microlitre of blood. "It wasn't anywhere near being low. So it wasn't a neutropenic fever. I emailed my oncologist, who emailed me back saying that we'll take care of things and figure it out, and if they can't figure it out they will contact me on Tuesday. But the fever broke and it has stayed down now. It's like 36.4, 36.7."

"So it's just one of those mysteries at the moment?"

"Yeah, I could always blame it on the chemotherapy, but it's going to be one of those mysteries that I'm not going to solve."

"How are you feeling today?"

"So far, so good. I was in bed almost all day yesterday. I got up for ten minutes. I had no appetite, I didn't drink much. I didn't eat much. I had a bit of supper and just collapsed in bed about 8:30 p.m. and then woke up this morning at 8:30 a.m. Other than getting up a couple times, as old men have to in the middle of the night, it was fine. I'm not totally energized but I'm better than I was yesterday. Yesterday I felt like someone had put a spigot in me and my energy all drained out of me. But it's coming back."

"So, this was the first chemo in this round?"

"Of three, supposedly … another three.… But I've never completed three. The oncologist says only twenty-five percent of people never complete three. He did reduce the dosage a bit this time, so we'll see whether that has an impact or not."

"So when are you due for your CT scan?"

"At the end of July. July 22."

"So you won't know until then what impact this has had…?"

"No … that's one of the things in deciding whether to have the CT scan … do I really want to know? There's advantage to not knowing, because I've got a little more knowledge than the average turkey out there, so if they say this node has increased in size … but another node has decreased in size, what does that mean? Well, it means nothing. Or if there's smaller liver mets, but more of them, it's … relating those things to the eventual outcome. Either prognosis is fraught with hazard. And I have warned patients against that. Oncologists are really good about scheduling CT scan after CT scan and watching the tumour grow and

I've done a couple extras where I have said, you know, once you see it grow, and you're not providing any more treatment that's effective, why would you want to know the size of it? Because unless you get into some problem that you can't predict anyways or do anything about, why would you want to know? I will go ahead because my family is interested. I'm not so interested. I would rather just feel better, or not feel better with the chemo and stop it. Make that the decision point rather than the tumour growth. But here I am … it will be three months after my diagnosis at the end of the week so it's … I'm still here. Which I didn't expect to be, after the first couple of weeks."

CHAPTER 17

Blockage

Canada Day, a day of bright sunshine. A day to be outside with your friends and your family. A day to enjoy that most ephemeral of things: the Canadian summer. A day that made little difference to Larry and me, or to our routine. He was hardly in any shape to be parading around in the sunshine, and our time together was limited. It had been ten days since our last meeting. I'd had a cold the previous week, so I'd stayed away. Larry's immune system was being wiped out by the chemo; a cold can be serious for a cancer patient. Since he was sequestered in his condo, that's where I needed to be too. Bella, Larry's PSW, had the day off, so it was just Faye, Larry, and me.

There was none of Larry's usual banter as I set up my recording equipment in his office. As I hauled the microphone and stand out of my bag, he asked about Natalie, about my son, who had visited Toronto the previous week, about my grandkids. He was, as always, polite and interested. But his trademark humour was absent.

He held a fan, a battery-operated hand-held model, and cycled it slowly, left to right, right to left, as he spoke. "I used to laugh about these things. Not anymore."

There was something almost distant in his tone. As if he were an onlooker, someone who had been pushed to the edge of the ring of life, someone who was no longer involved in its cut and thrust.

Today's topic was a subject that strains the imagination of the artist. A subject that's almost impossible to make fascinating or romantic: constipation.

The human bowel doesn't inspire great art. The scatological tends to the base or the juvenile. It's not a topic to lift the spirit and raise our consciousness to the consideration of the profound mysteries of life. But when something goes wrong with the bowel's silent workings, it quickly becomes our dominant obsession. It's all we can think about. The efficient and unconsidered work of the bowel is the very thing that frees us to consider weightier, more important things.

Because it's a problem commonly seen in palliative patients, Larry was something of an expert on constipation. It earned him the nickname the King of Constipation during his time as a palliative-care physician. So the irony of his being plagued by constipation was not lost on him.

"You know, we always joked that the anus controls the rest of the body when it's stopped up. Well, I can tell you, it does."

He sighed, leant forward. "My constipation hit me again this week. It is the worst. Of course, it's caused by the opiates, but it's also caused by one of the chemo drugs I'm taking. So I was in distress for two or three days. Two days ago they gave me an injection with a drug that was supposed to help, but it didn't. The nurses came back yesterday and gave me another shot, and it finally worked and it was like hallelujah! I should take pictures of this." He shook his head, laughed, but he was quick to erase the smile. This was serious stuff. "My bowels have become a source of anxiety for me. More than my pain. I'm less worried about my pain because I'm a pain physician and I know I've gone this far and it's not likely that my pain will get worse, unless I have some terrible end-stage problem and then I will be happily sedated."

The drug he used is called Relistor. It's the only medication specific to opioid-induced constipation. "It was developed by a pharmacologist at the University of Chicago who had cancer and who had terrible constipation. He said to himself that he should be able to design something in the lab to help him.*

---

* Larry's version of this story is slightly different from that published by the University of Chicago itself. According to the *University of Chicago Chronicle* (Vol. 19, No. 10, February 17, 2000) methylnaltrexone was developed by University of Chicago pharmacologist Leon Goldburg for a friend who had cancer and was suffering from morphine-induced constipation; http://chronicle.uchicago.edu/000217/drug.shtml.

"He started working with Naltrexone, which had been known for a while, but which isn't effective for patients on opioids because it crosses into the brain and makes them withdraw." The brain–blood barrier is a semi-permeable barrier that protects the brain from foreign substances in the blood that may damage the brain. Because it could cross this barrier, Naltrexone was able to block the action of the opioids that were relieving patients' pain. So it successfully treated the side effect, but in doing so it neutralized the drug.

"So he put a methyl-group molecule onto the Naltrexone, and lo and behold it didn't cross into the brain. So out of this work came a drug called Methylnaltrexone." The only problem with Methylnaltrexone is it doesn't cross the gut either, so it has to be given by injection.

Larry had history with this drug. He was one of the North American physicians who'd promoted it as an answer to constipation for some patients. He'd co-authored an article on it* and developed an education program with guidelines for its use. "It wasn't the first thing we recommended," he said. "We recommended other laxatives, and if they didn't work, we said try this."

He'd also been on the advisory board that made a pricing recommendation to the final licensee of the drug, Pfizer. "We said keep it around twelve to eighteen dollars a shot and you'll be able to sell this drug. Make it any higher in the Canadian market and you're not going to be able to sell it. Did they listen to us? No. They priced it at thirty dollars a shot. So the drug was reviewed by every drug review mechanism in every province, and the CDR [the Common Drug Review] told the provinces it didn't think they should accept the drug. So not a single province accepted Relistor.

"The only way you can get it is if you pay for it. But it's not only the cost of the drug and the needle, it's the nurse coming in to administer it. I went to buy some after I was discharged from Princess Margaret. It worked out at about forty dollars a shot."

And that's when things got complicated. Larry ran out of shots the previous week, so he called the pharmacy at Mount Sinai Hospital to buy some more. Bad news: the drug's distributor had withdrawn it in Canada because

* "Methylnaltrexone in the Treatment of Opioid-Induced Constipation in Cancer Patients Receiving Palliative Care: Willingness-to-Pay and Cost-Benefit Analysis," *Journal of Pain and Symptom Management*, Vol. 41, Issue 1, January 2011.

of poor sales. And they were out of stock. "Well, duh," Larry said, "we could've told you, you could've sold double the amount of the drug and more, and achieved the same profit, probably more, if you'd lowered the price. That's not the pharmaceutical industry's way. They price high while they hold the patents to recoup their research and development costs, which are immense for most drugs that hit the market today." Larry and his colleagues had reminded the manufacturer that the R&D costs on this drug were minimal. "This drug was probably the cheapest drug they've ever [made] because it was already researched, it was already developed. It's a simple chemical process. It's not an obtuse chemical antibody or anything like that."

Larry panicked. He'd tried other drugs for his constipation, "but it's the only thing that's been working consistently for my bowels. You know you become fixated … your head becomes up your asshole."

Fortunately, Larry had people in the U.S. He was a consultant at Northwest University in Chicago for years and had also filled a number of academic positions there. "It just so happened that a cousin from Chicago was visiting some cousins in Cleveland at the same time my mother-in-law was there. I called my folks in the States. I got a friend in Chicago to write a prescription for me. He gave it to my cousin, she took it to Cleveland, and my mother-in-law picked it up."

The hand-off was in Cleveland.

Larry couldn't suppress a smile at the thought of his mother-in-law, the drug mule, smuggling drugs across the border. "Fortunately the drug is registered in Canada, so it's not like it's an illegal drug. So she brought it home yesterday. I got the bill, and twenty-one boxes (shots) of the drug was fifteen hundred dollars, which was roughly seventy-five dollars a shot. Last time, when I bought it from Princess Margaret, it cost me about five hundred dollars, and our insurance paid eighty percent of that. So you wonder how anybody in the States ever affords it.

"But it finally worked yesterday, and I was so relieved. It gives you an idea of the cost. I'm willing to bear it, I mean if I need it. It's not like this is a forever drug."

He said it's further evidence of the short-sightedness of the pharmaceutical industry. "They're not interested in people. They're interested in profits and selling drugs and making enough R&D money for the next drug, so we're always paying.

"So that's the story of the drug and my bowels. Because my symptoms are part of that. My appetite. I wish my appetite were a bit better at times. You know, I love my ice cream and chocolate."

"And you're drinking coffee again ..."

"Yeah, I'm drinking coffee again. At least a cup of coffee a day. I can tolerate the coffee, usually in the morning. I'm trying to avoid too much juice. It's funny, cancer patients have always told me their taste changes. My tastes have changed. So I'll have a craving for something one week and I can't stand it the next. I'm still losing weight, which isn't a great sign. It's just the activity of the disease ... and then the nurse in the chemo unit says you're not drinking enough! Well, when you're nauseated and feeling shitty you don't feel like drinking. Guy! Put yourself in my shoes."

It was palpable, this sense of Larry as patient, a role he'd rarely had to play until now. And it's interesting, not so much the observation itself but the fact that a physician should be surprised that this is the world as it unfolds to the rest of us when we're in the hands of the health-care system. It cements my realization that most physicians (and even some nurses) are blithely and woefully unaware of the world as the patient sees it. A suspicion confirmed, in part at least, by what Larry said next.

"It's that failure again throughout the whole system to see the world as it occurs for the patient. So how can I drink more if I have enough trouble getting food past my teeth in the first place. Even plain water has a funny taste to it. Over the last couple of weeks I've had this salty taste that's partly the yeast infection in my mouth. It just varies. My taste varies, my food likes and dislikes vary. I like fruits and all the rest. They don't have a lot of calories in them so I try to have calorific fruits. I love soups, so Faye goes crazy trying to make me different kinds of soups. It drives my mother-in-law crazy when I don't eat. She tries her best to bring stuff that will make me feel better, but it doesn't work. So it's that craziness."

It's a theme we'd discussed before, of course, the importance of the ritual of celebration and companionship around food. Family and friends stand helpless on the sidelines, watch their loved one suffer the slash, poison, and burn ordeals of medical science. Food is something *they* can do. The practical palliative our loved ones *can* provide.

"Otherwise, the weakness comes and goes. Overall, I'm walking better. I only really need the cane just for some basic support if I'm going outside. I don't use it in here. I don't have any headaches. I don't have any visual disturbances …"

"And you don't seem to have any chemo fog today."

"No! Since they reduced the dosage it's made a big difference. It's the Paclitaxel that gives me the chemo fog. I've noticed that certainly with the Dexamethasone it puts you up high, but there isn't the same sort of coming down again … but yesterday was just one of those days that I was really down just because of the bad night before. The chemo fog seems to have dissipated though my memory … for what happened ten minutes ago … it's 'did I do that, or?' … 'did I take my medications, or?'… so that's what I still have some difficulty with. I really still want to get out each day. So if I don't get packed with visitors, to be able to go out and say I've done something in the day, even if it's been to go to Yorkdale and buy a pair of underwear, it's something. It's something to do, you know, go out and have some coffee with a friend. Those are the things that I need to do. I don't think I'm wasting my time. But I think I'm starting to get a bit bored. Partly because I think I surprised myself. I've lived longer than I thought I was going to live. So whatever is going on inside me, that nasty little tumour, as it eats its way through me … I guess I'll find out with the CT scan, but I'm not sure if it will tell me anything more about time. I'm not sure I want to know about time. It's again waking up every day and not knowing is this the first of the last of my days or did I gain another day? Is it one more day? Lord? Do you know? Help me, Lord, wherever the hell you are. Up, down, sideways.

"I have to meet with the rabbi again because I have some ideas about my funeral that I want to pass by her, since I want the funeral in the synagogue. Not that I am going to do anything gross and disgusting or severely anti-Jewish, but there are some things that I would like to have done which probably some of my relatives will think, 'Oy! He really was crazy!'"

That seemed a good point to close the discussion. I packed my recording equipment away and headed for the ravine. It was one of those days when I needed to think. Larry's concern about his wasted time, his need to do something tangible with his day, resonated with me for two reasons.

The first was my own health-care issues six years before — a heart attack that changed my life's perspectives and priorities.

The second was the request Larry had asked of me just before I packed up my equipment.

CHAPTER 18

Walk

I was sitting on a toilet in the basement of a shabby pub on the Danforth, having what may have been a heart attack, and the first thought to hit me was, *Damn, I'm going to die like Elvis.* Well, not exactly like Elvis. I was dressed in a football strip, and I wasn't in a fabulous mansion.

I'd always pictured a heart attack as sudden, and much more painful, the way it is in movies: victim falls to the floor, face twisted in agony, clutches his heart. This just felt like displaced indigestion. No wonder people ignore it and end up dead on the toilet.

If I had to die like a rock star I'd rather it wasn't Elvis. But then, which rock star dies an elegant, decorous death? Not John Bonham. He choked to death on his own vomit. Certainly not John Lennon, shot by a random nutcase looking for fifteen minutes of fame. I would rather have lived like a rock star and died like an accountant: a quiet, comfortable, suburban death. Instead, it seemed I'd lived like an accountant and was dying like a bloated, overweight rock star.

Maybe it wasn't a heart attack. I pulled up my shorts and climbed the stairs to the bar where the rest of my recreational football team waited.

It was Monday, June 14, 2007 — the beginning of Natalie's second week at the Latner Centre. She'd gone there principally because of her new boss's reputation. It was a not-to-be-missed opportunity, working with the celebrated Dr. Librach.

By the time I got back to the bar, our captain, Pete, had ordered pitchers, nachos, and wings. I wished I felt like beer — a bad sign. I reached for a glass and poured a tumbler of water. I chugged a few mouthfuls, strained water through ice, hoped it would ease the burning.

I felt my pulse. My heart was still beating. That was a comfort. What did I expect to feel in the throb of my wrist? S.O.S tapped out in Morse code by my ailing heart? *Fool.*

Now I was clammy. A cold sweat, one of the signs. I would have to make a decision soon. I couldn't sit there having a heart attack all evening. What if it turned out to be indigestion after all? I'd feel like an idiot. On the other hand, I'd look idiotic if I ignored it and ended up dead. What was the statistic? Fifty percent of all heart attacks are fatal? Those were not good odds.

The beer showed up. Pete was about to pour a round. As an Englishman I couldn't allow a pint to be wasted. It was time to make a decision. I pulled myself to my feet. My legs seemed to have filled with sand in the five minutes since I sat down. The discomfort in my chest had swelled, felt more like pressure than acid burn. Around the table, heads turned. This was unprecedented. I was leaving as the beer arrived. "I have to go," I said. "I don't feel well. Colin, can I get my stuff from your car?"

Colin had driven me to the bar from the field. My boots and street clothes were still in his trunk. Maybe I'd get a cab home. Maybe I'd go straight to the hospital. I'd see how I felt. We started to weave through the bar together, but I could barely walk. I felt weighty, tugged downward by a sudden increase in gravity. I was short of breath. I'd just played a full game of football — two halves of thirty-five minutes each — and scored three goals. Now I couldn't walk?

"Are you okay?" Colin asked. "You want me to drive you to the hospital?"

"I don't know. I don't think I can walk to the car. Where is it?"

"Around the corner."

"I don't think I can walk any farther. Maybe I'll get a cab."

"Are you sure? I can drive you to the hospital."

I hesitated. I'd already dragged him away from beer, I didn't want to ruin his entire evening. Bands of pain tightened around my chest.

"Yeah, maybe you should."

"You wait here. I'll bring the car around."

Colin was a drug rep. He must have been adding it all up: chest pains, shortness of breath, clammy skin. He probably knew what was happening.

I knew what was happening. Neither of us dared mention it. He disappeared over the road. I slumped against a lamppost. There was a bistro next to the pub. The patio waitress, lean and blond and dressed in undertaker black, looked over at me. Was that concern behind her eyes, or did she think I was drunk?

"Are you okay? Would you like a drink of water?"

"I just had some. I'm fine." In England anyone who isn't actually dead is fine. I was just having a heart attack.

The pain was getting worse, like my heart was being crushed. How did people ignore this? I bent down, worried I wouldn't be able to stand again when Colin arrived. Maybe we should have called an ambulance. It was too late now. Couldn't change my mind when I'd made someone give up their parking spot, not in this neighbourhood.

The iron bands around my chest tightened another notch. I started to feel dizzy with the pain.

Colin swung his car across four lanes of busy Danforth traffic to universal disgust and a couple of angry horns. He jumped out to help me into the passenger seat, but I waved him away. As long as I could move independently I couldn't be dying.

I climbed in and leant against the window, spent. The pain had now become a pressure. Like someone had laid a large stone on my chest. Colin headed south. "Do you want to call Nat?" She hates being called Nat. If you have to call her anything but Natalie, call her Nal. I didn't call her Nal. She'd always been Natalie to me. Always would be. Always. Always isn't always as long as we would like it to be.

He offered me his mobile. My glasses were in my bag, which was on the back seat. I didn't have the strength to fish them out, so I squinted and punched.

"Hello?" She was hesitant, a query in her tone. Of course, she didn't recognize Colin's number.

"Hi."

"Oh, hi," she said, suddenly breezy. She probably thought I'd cut beers with the team so we could meet on the patio of our local, The Jason George, for a beer. I drew a breath. I had to sound calm. Like this was just routine. "I don't feel well. Colin's driving me to the hospital."

"What's up?"

"I have a pain in my chest, and I'm short of breath."

"Oh, sweetie." Her voice scoured flat, her words suddenly grey, monotone, lifeless. "I'll see you at the hospital. I'll meet you there." She used to work at Heart and Stroke. She knew.

Still, it wasn't indigestion, which was a relief. At least I wouldn't look like an idiot.

Boxes of meds littered the back seat of Colin's car. There was probably enough aspirin to raise Elvis. Neither of us thought to put a tablet under my tongue, like the public awareness campaigns tell you to.

Unaccountably, he kept stopping. I wanted to scream. Didn't he know I was in pain? He tried to reassure me: "It's OK. Almost there. Just a few minutes." Who put in all these traffic lights? Must they all be red?

It took twenty minutes to reach St. Mike's Hospital. Colin wanted to help me up the ramp, but I waved him away. It was the usual turmoil inside Emerge. People on gurneys, people on crutches, people with bloody bandages, children crying. At the entrance, three or four paramedics chatted, a stack of pizza boxes in their arms. Business as usual.

Natalie was not there yet. I walked over to a grubby orange vinyl hospital seat, one of the hard plastic injection moulded ones, and subsided into it. Now everything was in the hands of professionals. Except it wasn't. Colin wandered from station to station, looped back and forward, tried to find help. I thought about staging a collapse to get some attention, because Colin had been told, once again, to sit and wait. I closed my eyes. Everything got a little more blurry, a little less real. I retreated to some other place. Somewhere inside my head. The pain was now so intense I didn't really care if I lived or died. I was not frightened. I just wanted someone to give me enough painkillers to make it stop, or to kill me.

I realized with a shock I didn't tell Natalie where Colin was taking me. But then Natalie was there. She screamed, "My husband is having a heart attack!" Nobody had dared mention it till then. My secret was out. The elephant in the room stumbled over to my corner and sat on my chest. I curled around the pain as if nursing it, my body folded around it like a salted slug.

Nevertheless, the grim-faced triage nurse behind her glass partition wanted me to walk over to her kiosk. I stood, and shuffled over there. I was still in my football strip, wearing a pair of street shoes, loafers. A fashion faux pas I found embarrassing, even in such extremis.

I could barely speak. She fired off a quick burst of questions. She couldn't wait to reload, so I answered fast at first, but the world retreated behind the pain, and my voice trailed away.

"Sir, I need you to sit up straight and speak clearly," she barked. Normally, I'm compliant, but for once I didn't care what she needed. I had my own needs: principally the need to concentrate on bearing the pain. Natalie took over, answered her questions. I slipped into Painland.

I was wheeled away. As I passed through the beige curtains that separated triage from the waiting room I entered a parallel universe where time is king. On the other side of the curtains, time did not matter. Here time was your ally. It saved lives. How these universes could coexist without destroying each other baffled me. I climbed onto the gurney.

I felt like a sugar lump, fallen too close to an anthill. Busy hands swarmed over me. A nurse leant in to break the news. "You've come to the right place." I was grateful for her observation — I was comforted to be told I'd made the right decision — but felt I didn't deserve her praise. It seemed the obvious place to come when you're having a heart attack. "You're in good hands." Excellent. I was starting to worry about that in the waiting room. And now the big one. "You're having a heart attack."

"I know. If I wasn't, I'd still be in the bar." What sane person chooses an emergency room over a bar?

Natalie was ushered into a waiting room while they worked on me. After twenty minutes of torture, alone in a darkened room, a nurse delivered the news to her. "Your husband is having a myocardial infarction."

"Thank God. I thought he was having a heart attack."

They gave me aspirin. Swedish men are told to carry a tablet in their wallet. I pictured a heart-attack victim flapping around on a Stockholm sidewalk like a beached salmon, while passersby frisked him. Looks of horror on tourists' faces. A callous nation, the Swedes.

They sprayed me under the tongue with nitroglycerin. They gave me morphine, hooked me up to a couple of IV lines. Now they asked me about my habits. They were concerned I may have abused drugs. "Not until I got here," I told them.

Slowly, too slowly, the pain receded. The world came back into focus. Things calmed down. There was less swarming. Natalie arrived, red-eyed.

"You've been crying," I said. It wasn't an observation, it was an apology. I hadn't intended pain.

A young doctor leant over the gurney, a day's growth of stubble on his chin, his shirt and white coat crumpled as if they'd been slept in, not necessarily by him. He wore a pair of grubby trainers whose laces trailed on the floor. There were bags under his eyes. I was tempted to offer him my gurney. He looked as if he needed it more than me. He told me I had been given a clot-busting drug, to clear my blocked artery. If it didn't work, they would have to intervene. It wasn't clear what that meant and he didn't explain. Would it entail rib spreading, I wondered?

I'd have asked, but it didn't seem to matter that much. I was touched and a little amused by the concern of the doctor and nurses. They took everything too seriously. They needed to chill out. No wonder doctors burnt out young. The morphine had kicked in.

There was nothing to do but wait for the clot buster. They moved me to the cardiac ward. If the clot wasn't busted in forty minutes they said, they'd intervene. The pain had backed off a little. The elephant was up and parading around the room, but there was still a large rock on my chest, so I was given more morphine. I was more tired than I'd ever been.

At five minutes past intervention time the rock on my chest melted away. Almost immediately a nurse was in the room, ready to intervene. But my clot had been busted.

Natalie sat by my bed while I slept, watched me, the clock, the array of instruments over the bed. Willed my heart not to stop. Around 4 a.m. I woke. I felt almost normal. I looked up. Natalie lifted her head and peered through the darkness, into my eyes. "I feel better," I said. "Can we go home now?"

Elvis had left the building.

Natalie and I went for a long walk on the Saturday following my Canada Day discussion with Larry. The pretext was a new bag. Mine was falling apart. The bag I wanted, a *faux* antique CBC canvas bag, was stocked by a number of shops in Toronto a couple of years previously, but not anymore. The manufacturer's showroom was a six-kilometre walk, but I was grateful for it. I felt as if I had something large and muscular coiled within me: something that had been growing there since I started this journey with Larry, and I hoped the walk would exorcise it.

Natalie was quiet at first. I was grateful for that. It was a hot day. The humidity had finally caught up with the city after a cold, wet start to the summer, and I was sweating pretty generously. But then the subject of Larry came up. Our session had been quite a rough one and I'd been quiet about it since. I didn't share how low Larry seemed. How lost.

She didn't skirt the question. Just asked me straight out: "How are you feeling about the Larry thing now?" So there it was, sitting steaming on the sidewalk in front of me.

The Larry thing? What exactly was the Larry thing? During our last conversation Larry had raised a new question. In the space of a week, three people in "reasonably high places" had told him he should write a book to capture his experiences of the cancer system from the patient side: his thoughts about it, and about how we die. He said he was flattered and energized by the idea, but he said, "I don't think I can write a book. I mean, I've got ideas about what a book might look like, and I've got ideas about how it would differ from what you're doing, or could incorporate what you are doing. But could I write a book? No. It's not what I intended to do. But when the head of oncology at Princess Margaret says you've got to write a book, and when Dr. Marla Shapiro says the same thing, you have to take notice."

What would that do to my project, the article I was planning? I had no idea, but I thought it would probably bury it. How would it work? Larry was clear he didn't want a ghost writer. He saw us as co-authors of this book. We'd kicked the idea around for half an hour or so, and it was clear to me that neither of us really knew exactly what a book might look like.

The most important factor was that we shared a passion for the subject, and a similar drive to advance the cause of end-of-life care. I'd told him I'd help him with this last task. He'd finished the memory boxes for his grandchildren, got his financial affairs in order, and had admitted, "I'm frankly getting bored. So the opportunity to dictate some ideas into Dragon Speak [a voice-recognition program]... I can put myself to work, at least a couple of hours a day on that."

I understood his impulse to tell his story. Lying in a hospital bed six years previously, I'd made a somewhat similar determination: to take my writing more seriously and dedicate full attention and effort to it. Brushes with death tend to focus us that way. This was something Larry needed to do before his time ran out.

"I'd love to help you," I said, "because I think the people you spoke to are absolutely right. You do have something very valuable to say. There's an openness and an honesty that you bring to the subject which is difficult to find."

So that was the Larry Thing. I was used to things taking sudden turns (for the worse, or better). Anyone who's lived long and widely is used to it. But this request of Larry's had me knotted and tied. To begin with, he was relying on me to get this story out. I'd be responsible for it, answerable if I failed. I wasn't used to that. I was used to being responsible only to myself in my writing. Used to being the only one I could let down. But it wasn't just that.

I tried to explain the problem to Natalie. "I knew this was going to be hard. I'm trying to maintain a professional poise with Larry, but it's becoming next to impossible to do. Every time I see him he's a little weaker. A little less Larry. He's still substantially Larry, but I can see his light fading, visit by visit. It's tough to watch."

What I didn't tell her was that I'd caught myself indulging in the kind of silly fantasies that caregivers often fall prey to: the hope for a sudden miracle cure, emerging from a lab in the U.S. or Europe, a miracle (an even more unlikely outcome) of a religious nature perhaps. I'd begun to ask myself what I'd do if I had just one wish. I would ask for Larry to be cured. The world needs more Larrys. It wasn't fair he should be die before his race was fully run. I realized I'd crossed the line.

Let's be honest, there is no line. There's an idea of a line. Not even that. The thought of the idea of a line. Wherever it was, I'd crossed it sometime before without noticing. Did that make me more or less useful as Larry's co-author, if that was what I was now meant to be? Writers of fiction know they must get inside their characters. They must know them through and through, feel their griefs and their jubilations, care about them. If this is true of fiction, why shouldn't it also be true of non-fiction? Could a growing intimacy with, and affection for, Larry be a bad thing? The wrong thing?

Then I remembered something else. Writers of fiction sometimes care too much for their characters. They flinch, because they want to save them the hardest trials.

This was what I was wanting for Larry. I wanted to spare him. I was flinching. That wasn't what he needed from me. He needed me to not flinch, to complete the journey with him. By his side. Every step.

We were due to meet again on Monday, July 8. On Sunday, July 7, Faye emailed me to cancel. Larry had a low-grade fever and his oncologist had called him in. Larry wrote to me later that day: "Sorry about cancelling this morning but had to see the oncologist urgently. We are stopping the chemo because all indicators point to the fact that it is not working. My weakness is increasing fairly rapidly. Bound and determined to finish our project."

CHAPTER 19

Stoic

We normally eased into our talks together gently, while I got the mike set up, tested the levels, and Faye or Bella organized a coffee. Today was different. Larry was quiet. He waited until I was ready, although he seemed to bristle with anticipation. He had some news for me. As soon as I hit record it spilled out.

"Yesterday was the first day in about five days where I felt like I could do something. No chemo. No chemo, no, sir. So I'm in a different phase of my illness. It's interesting the way people have taken this decision."

Throughout his chemo journey Larry was always slightly frustrated by the assumption that since he'd submitted to chemo he hoped for a cure. He explained, frequently yet patiently, that the chemo was to help manage his symptoms and perhaps extend his life for a few weeks or months. It wasn't an attempt to cure him. Even so, some of his circle continued to urge him to fight the cancer, to persevere, try to beat it: an enterprise the odds didn't favour. But the decision to stop wasn't his, which was a relief.

"It was made by the oncologist. I went into the meeting with a sense that I didn't want to continue the chemo, but he really brought it forward, which I thought was really good for Faye to hear because she wasn't quite sure. I've had increasing problems with the chemo. Sure it's nice to be manic when you have the Decadron, but otherwise … Sunday and Monday were miserable days. Monday, in particular, I was just beside myself. Couldn't make hide nor hair of things, and then Tuesday wasn't much better."

Today was, unusually, a Thursday. Unusual because we normally met on Mondays and Fridays. "But it was mostly GI complaints. I couldn't depend on the chemo to do one thing … either it makes me constipated or it gives me diarrhea. It gave me both. So you figure it out. It was just sapping energy from me. Then I realized I spent a day and a half a week, at least, in chemo. It was a day of chemo and half a day around blood tests and worrying about who was going to take me down, and what are the counts now … it was draining on me. I didn't see any benefit. The early benefit I saw was some gain in energy. It was real but it's disappeared."

We sat in Larry's office, which doubled as a bedroom when necessary. It was a small but comfortable room, with his desk set against the wall, on the opposite side of the room to the window. He sat in one of those leather-clad office chairs, the kind that rests on a halo — easy to spin on but hard to shift to and fro. He spun around to look for something, spun back again. "I've also noticed this past couple of weeks what we call proximal myopathy" — he ran his hands over his thighs — "where my muscles, my big muscles that hold me upright and the muscles of my arm" — he lifted his arm, grasped his tricep with his other hand — "are shrinking away at an enormously quick rate and it's not just from disuse. It's really an effect of the disease. The muscles literally melt away and the Decadron contributes to that. So I find it difficult to get out of the chair. Like the chair I'm sitting in today, I have to push up with my arms in order to get out." He demonstrated. His elbows shook a little as he strained to push himself to his feet. It was hard to resist the instinct to get up and help him. "Normally I should be able to stand without using my arms. Not long ago I could have got up with my arms crossed in front of me." He shook his arms, as if he was shaking away the effort, then gently let himself fall back into the chair.

"There comes a time, too, and it's been harder to describe to people. I spoke to David Kendal [about it] yesterday, because he and I have seen this in patients before. The patient becomes aware their body is failing them totally. I know my body is failing me. And it's failing me because of the cancer. It's not because I don't try or don't eat. It's the cancer advancing. That's supported by my tumour markers — they've started to go up again. They went down for a while and now they are back up, so … that indicates the tumour … the chance of response, like a significant response, was low anyways, but this just means there was no response. Which made decision-making quite easy."

Larry hadn't used his portable fan today, but the effort of talking clearly overheated him. He pulled a linen handkerchief from his pocket and wiped the sweat from his forehead. "Hang on a minute, let me go and get that blessed fan."

I knew Larry's decision would cause some ripples amongst the people closest to him. When considered dispassionately, and knowing Larry's priorities — that he remain mentally alert and present for as long as possible while controlling his symptoms — it was the right decision. But there was a finality to it too. As if an unlikely escape hatch had just closed for good. I asked if he'd had any backlash against the decision, anyone who thought he'd given up?

"Some people saw it as giving up. I've caught that in conversations with people … you know, you're giving up, you should still try, and that kind of thing. Others have supported it. Certainly my family supported it: Faye … and the kids …"

This was significant for Larry, and the main reason he was grateful his oncologist had made the decision for him. He had only been able to guide them so far down the road of acceptance. It seemed they'd been helped to that final step by Larry's doctor.

"I haven't told my mother-in-law yet. I'm not sure I want to." Larry loved his mother-in-law. It was evident in his expression, and in the way he spoke of her. His reticence was born of compassion.

"Do you think she'll take that view that you've given up?"

"I think so. Although in one conversation recently she indicated that she had backed off from her position that I was going to live forever … seemed to recognize that I was dying. I know there are some friends who are physicians who see the chemo … I've got to take it … I've got no choice. But this here body ain't listening to them or the chemotherapies. Enough is enough. So it's been hard for me. From the point of view of, okay, so now what?"

That was the big question. If the chemo made things worse, why continue? To placate friends and family? Just to have something to do, to feel as if you've at least tried? Even if you know, intellectually, that it's pointless, it's difficult to do nothing.

"My fears are still there, and the fear of the end, not the fear of getting to the end but the fear of what the end means. The fear of making sure that nothing goes terribly awry, so that my family doesn't have to see me suffer intolerably. Those are still there. And also, what does it mean for me? You know, I finished the memory boxes. I just have to print up the letters today and then the boxes will be delivered. They're all set. I've written a little speech for my funeral, which I want to make sure the rabbi is okay with. It doesn't castigate anybody. It's really just thanking people for being part of my life. I've never seen that at a Jewish funeral, but they are about to get one. There is a prescribed nature to a Jewish funeral, but I've always tilted against windmills a little bit. I don't mind doing that. And you know, can we finish the book in time? It's really my only project now. And I really want to get to work on that."

It was a good question. In the two months since we started I'd accumulated a lot of material. But we hadn't yet fleshed out what had now become, to Larry, The Book. I didn't know, at that point, how much work he envisaged doing on The Book, how much material he'd already written in his own journal. And, crucially, I didn't know how much time we had. Nobody did. Not knowing the answer to any of these questions, I deflected, though I hardly realized I was doing so.

"And what will it mean physically, now you're in this phase of your illness?"

"It's a different experience for the elderly — now I have to consider myself the elderly. The great burden on the health-care system. I'll be more burdensome, as time goes on. We are looking at equipment we'll need here and whether we'll have to hire more help at some point. I told Faye very clearly she has to let me know when she feels she's being overwhelmed. But I don't need physical care at the moment, although Bella is very capable of doing the physical care as well as vacuuming. I'll need the physical care at some point. I've got a walker now because sometimes I feel unsteady. I've got the wheelchair, I've got the cane."

He still seemed fairly mobile, although the proximal myopathy was making it more challenging for him to get out of the condo.

"You're still able to get out and about?"

"I haven't been out for almost a week now. That's been the problem. Well, I shouldn't say that. Monday we went out because we went to the chemotherapy clinic. I went to the GI clinic. I had lunch with Dr. Yves Talbot and his wife. Saying goodbye to them, because they are going away on a trip … two cruises for twenty-three days. When you are saying goodbye it's very bittersweet, because I don't know if they will be here. I just don't know. The time … is really starting to pressure me. On the other hand I can't … there's a limit to what I can do in that time."

"David [Kendal] came see you yesterday. How did that go?"

"It went very well. He's going away for three or four weeks as well, at the end of July. Albert Kirshen will probably take over as the primary physician. I don't want to put too much pressure on Russell. David's very supportive. He's really good at assessing a home, whether it's adequate for maintaining somebody in a home-care environment. My home-care coordinator is on vacation as well. When she comes back she will come in to assess that as well.

"It's interesting, the nurses want to increase the number of visits to three times a week, which I see as totally unnecessary. To be honest with you, because I need those injections, I didn't put up a huge fight about it, but I said I could always cancel one if I didn't need it. I think they want to do it because they learn so much from me about palliative care. I was telling one of them the other day about my weakness, the proximal myopathy. She said, 'I didn't realize' ... said she'd have to look that up. She's probably seen it about ten dozen times in her patients. She just didn't recognize it. That has a big impact, of course, on whether people can be mobile.

"But it's been interesting, their reaction to all this. I guess it's a symbol of my value to them, but it's really totally unwarranted at the moment."

"Touching, though."

"Yes, it is. They just want to look after me. So either I'm a big, huggable teddy bear, or they are afraid of doing something wrong."

I wondered if there was anything else he wanted to get done. I couldn't quite get the words "before you die" out. But they were there in the unbroken silence that hung in the room for a second while he thought.

"I want to try to make it up to the cottage. That's the one missing piece. Would I regret not making it up to the cottage? Yes. But if I can't make it up to the cottage, I can't make it up to the cottage. There is a limit to ... the risks are ... once next week rolls around, when my counts will stabilize and start going up if they haven't started already going up, then I can probably take a couple days and say goodbye to the cottage, and talk to my wife and son about what needs to be done so they can sell it ... I'll just have to see the way it goes. That's my one little regret. I don't really have others. I'm sure I would have liked to see the new Superman movie or whatever, but those don't enter into the reality of my situation."

Larry had always been an avid consumer of popular culture. When *Avatar* was released in 2009 he was enchanted with it, in all its three-dimensional glory, and had insisted that Natalie had to see it too. If there was a new gadget to be purchased, a smartphone, or a tablet, Larry was likely to be at the front of the queue. But after his diagnosis he found his perspective shifted.

"I find watching TV and reading the newspaper … a lot of the stuff that's going on doesn't mean a wit to me…. I'm dying …who cares about who's dumping who … the stars, the celebrities …why are we worrying about this? We should be worrying about important things: train safety, the fact that the bees are all dying … there's so much news that's not news."

His point was not, I think, that these distractions are per se bad, not even that they are worthless, just that, if we allow them to they will distract us from the real, the essential, components of our lives. It reminded me of an adage I'd grappled with in my late teenage years.

Apparently it was Marcus Aurelius who told us we should live every day as if it were our last. What he actually said was: "To live each day as though one's last, never flustered, never apathetic, never attitudinizing — here is perfection of character." When I first stumbled across this quote (it's in volume seven of Aurelius's *Meditations*) at eighteen, I found it intimidating and a touch absurd.

Of course, I understood the whole *carpe diem* idea. Life is finite. Make the most of it. But it didn't seem to take into account that in the modern world (and at eighteen years of age) the balance of probabilities are heavily stacked against Marcus's proposition.

It's an approach that may have served Roman emperors well, but they were (with some notable exceptions) a stoic bunch, with high moral standards and iron self-discipline. To a Roman such a tenet was a call to get a grip and live up to the standards of your ancestors. I can't shake the suspicion that we no longer remember the last half of the quote because it's out of tune with a hedonistic spin that's more amenable to our modern minds. We're prone to interpret Marcus's injunction as a pretext for abandonment. If today is your last day on Earth you don't need to worry about consequences. You can smoke as many cigarettes, drink as much alcohol, take as many drugs as you want. You won't be around to deal with the fallout. Why bother exercising self-control, why bother with moral codes, why worry about tomorrow if there is no tomorrow?

That's one way to look at it, but it's a perspective that's only possible in the Western world, and it's only been remotely feasible since the modern era. Since our species decided to settle down and grow our food, we've had to plan for the future. And for most of our agrarian history the vast majority of the population was involved in food production. If you didn't worry about tomorrow you'd starve. This was true even in Rome, and especially for the emperor, who had to feed his vast empire.

Since Aurelius's day we've devoted a lot of thought to the subject of planning for a future we've been increasingly able to control. Aurelius didn't have to worry about his pension (although the soldiers in his legions did) and he couldn't buy life insurance (or chariot coverage). Even so, when you've conquered the entire known world, the practical consequence is the need to plan efficiently. He had roads and aqueducts to build, legions to feed, arm, and stock, navies to equip. Though he was emperor, Aurelius couldn't afford to live a nihilistic existence of self-gratification. Not without destroying everything his ancestors had built. So he clearly couldn't have meant for his aphorism to be taken as a creed of Epicurian excess.

What was he saying then, if it was not that we should live recklessly, as if there were no consequences? He was saying we should live well, live fully, live to make a difference, an impact, a contribution. Since life is fleeting, we must make each day count. As much as we've extended life expectancy to almost double that of our forebears in Roman times, and as much as we try to avoid the simple certainty of our own end, we will all eventually have to face facts. Our lives are finite.

Larry's much more so. I wondered how he coped with that — the insistent countdown that ate away his remaining time. I wondered what he thought of Aurelius's maxim.

"I think it would be pretty difficult if I woke up every morning thinking that day could be my last. I think it would paralyze me more than it would help me. I always figure, keep an eye on a horizon. If you'd spoken to me the week after I was diagnosed, when I had all those problems, I didn't think I'd make it a week after that. So I take it a milestone at a time. I made it to my birthday, then after that Father's Day. What's the next milestone? There's really nothing until our wedding anniversary in August. That seems pretty far away to me."

I could see how this approach would help. But I still wondered how he kept himself protected from the mental anguish of the knowledge that time was rapidly running out. "Doesn't the idea that you can feel the breath of your pursuer on your neck, doesn't that get to you?" I asked.

"You can only get done today what you can get done today. I look at it in that way. I always try to plan some event, or have a visitor, or do something so I don't dwell on it. I can't allow myself to wonder if the next guy at the door will be the guy with the sickle over his shoulder and black robe."

Besides, he said, his body was already reminding him of his mortality. "When I get up every morning my back tells me I'm getting older. But as you grow older you start to develop a different view of things. And of course my career made me very cognizant of dying and death and the finite nature of life. Then my body told me a lot about how finite my resources were."

I'd heard the same thing from the other physicians at the Latner Centre. Their job is a daily reminder of our mortality. It changes the way they live their lives. I mentioned this to Larry.

"It does. You can't work in the business I worked in without being changed. Although now some people have started to medicalize things. I think there's a danger of us [palliative-care physicians] medicalizing death. If you talk to some of my younger colleagues, they don't have the broad experience of medicine and life yet, so I think a lot of them still are into [dealing with] symptoms. That's the thing they focus on: 'We're pain and symptoms.' When you see them work they cover the rest of it, but they see themselves almost as symptomatologists. They forget the people issues that they need to deal with."

What was Larry's worry? That they were ignoring the people issues altogether (issues like depression, pushing family and loved ones away, the increasing sense of isolation that can become acute as death approaches) or that they aren't quite getting the balance right, between dealing with the patient's symptoms and dealing with their psychological pain? "It's balance. Should they put as much focus on people issues when they visit as they put into adjusting pain medications, for example."

He also worried there's far too much investigation of end-of-life patients. "We do it just in case there's something we can correct. You know, putting an eighty-eight-year-old woman on antibiotics because she might have pneumonia, sending her for an X-ray. Well she had advanced cancer. As it turned out she didn't have pneumonia, but she was kept on the antibiotics. Well, why? There's no reason. She probably just caught an ordinary cold. And that's where medicine places us. That's why palliative-care physicians have always been a bit on the outs with medicine."

He leant back again, rubbed the end of his nose with his knuckle. He'd taken us back to the big picture again, the bigger issue, but I wasn't sure I'd got the answer to my question yet. How did he cope with the ever-present consciousness of his own mortality? We are all confronted with it at some point in our lives. Normally, when it happens, it overwhelms us. How was it not overwhelming Larry?

"Ninety percent of us will die with one or more chronic illnesses — that's the reality of things as you age. And it starts you thinking, yeah, sure I've got the pain, but dying is not the alternative I'd wish for. I wouldn't consider myself old. I just turned sixty-seven. I don't think that's old. But my body had started to inflict a variety of aches and pains on me. My hair was getting greyer and thinner. I couldn't do as much as I used to be able to do. The Boost couple on TV can go out, take a can of Boost, and play soccer with their grandkids. I can't.

"Of course life is finite, but I don't think of it like that. I don't think we're a death-denying society. We just like to put it aside, but if you look at TV now you see a lot more elderly people dying, rather than people just being gunned down or falling out of airplanes. So I think concepts are changing. We're seeing more in the newspapers about dying and death now. I think society is looking at it differently. The discussion on assisted death has probably helped."

I thought about that for a moment. Perhaps he was right. Perhaps we are, as a society, coming to grips with death, beginning to allow ourselves to take a long, steady look at it. In his book *A Social History of Dying*, Allan Kellehear challenged one of the most popular quotations about death: "One can look directly neither at the sun nor death." Kellehear calls Rochefoucauld's quote "tiresome and over-employed," and points out that "near-death studies, hospice and palliative-care research, as well as bereavement studies" mean we can now stare death in the face.

So why is it we still tidy away the old and the infirm into nursing homes? So we don't have to be disturbed or inconvenienced by their presence in our lives? I wondered aloud to Larry about the plight of the elderly. Doesn't that argue against his point? He agreed. "If you look at the conditions inside our nursing homes, they're just as bad as the way we treat our Native populations. You visit these places, nobody wants to be there, but sixteen percent of us in Ontario are going to die in a long-term care facility under abysmal conditions. They're like the residential schools. We pay so little to these long-term care facilities, but on the other hand they deliver so little."

It seemed a sombre note to end on, but perhaps an apt one. But as I started to tidy away my equipment, Larry couldn't resist a final foray into the big question of the day.

"I'm sure your experiences with your heart placed the finiteness of life in some kind of context. Scared the hell out of you."

"It made me reorder my priorities and decide what I wanted to do with the rest of my life for sure."

"Probably made you think that bucket list needed to be started earlier? I can't tell you how many people I watched die saying 'God I wish I'd travelled before.' You know, they save up for it, but never manage to do it."

Natalie's father had done the same thing. He worked hard to retire because he wanted to travel. He couldn't wait to retire, but he died before he was able to.

"So you just never know. We've always made travel a priority, because I always had a wanderlust. I've been able to do it, and had the money to do it. But I don't even think it needs a lot of money. How many people in this city have never been out of Ontario? Or Toronto, for that matter. I think more people should be making the choice to have that balance.

"I worked bloody hard, but I also played bloody hard, not at doing crazy things, but I had my family at the cottage, we travelled, I enjoyed myself when we travelled. We didn't have a lavish lifestyle. Palliative care led me to that balance so that now I could quit my jobs. They're not that important."

It didn't strike me until later, the subtle irony of that statement. Because while it was true Larry had walked away from his two jobs very easily, he hadn't given up his work. He still met with me, still taught his nurses about his condition, still trained his colleagues at the Latner Centre, never missed an opportunity to teach. I'm positive he didn't see the irony. His work was so deeply enmeshed in his character by then that it was one with everything he did.

In his last months and days he was able to clear the clutter away from his life, and what that left was plain to see: his family on the one hand, and his work on the other. Dying had stripped away everything else, shown them up for what they always were: superficialities. He achieved an enviable clarity. He seemed to be at peace with it.

CHAPTER 20

Hope

On Wednesday, July 17, Larry called in the morning to tell me he was on the front page of the *National Post*. A story about assisted death. The reporter, Tom Blackwell, had called because, in Larry's role as head of the University of Toronto's Joint Centre for Bioethics, he'd developed a program to teach health professionals how to deal with assisted-death requests. Blackwell didn't know Larry was dying. Larry, as ever, was perfectly frank about it. Blackwell got his story, and rang off.

Toward the end of the day he called Larry back. He'd filed his story, in which he had mentioned Larry's disease and prognosis. His editor asked him a question that was perhaps obvious, but difficult to address to a dying man: what about Larry? Now that he was dying, how did he feel about assisted death? I can understand why Tom Blackwell didn't ask this question initially. We're social animals and it's a distinctly antisocial question. Even a hardened journalist found it difficult to confront the starkness of Larry's death sentence.

But his editor made him call Larry back to ask the question. I imagine he was squirming inside as he picked up the phone. He probably felt like a callous jerk. As did I at times, many times, throughout this process. Because sometimes the very question you need to ask is the question that's the most difficult to face.

Why? Because I was worried that I might upset Larry? That he might, to the embarrassment of us both, dissolve in tears? Not really. He'd always been completely open with me, but had managed to retain his poise whenever we spoke. Although, of course, I knew he wasn't afraid to cry when he was alone with Faye, because he'd told me so. Perhaps it was because I might offend him, make him close up or kick me out altogether? That wasn't it either. It never happened, but I imagine if I'd asked him a question that was too intrusive he would have politely told me that was none of my business and moved on.

So none of the above. I think the problem lay in me. My benchmarks for the insensitive and offensive needed to be recalibrated. These were extraordinary circumstances, and Larry was uncommonly honest. I was consistently shocked by his willingness to open up to me.

On my way home from the gym that evening I picked up a copy of the newspaper from my local Metro. When I got home I opened up the paper and read Blackwell's story while I drank my daily Starbucks.

He opened the piece with a three-paragraph précis of one of the cases that changed Larry's mind on the issue of assisted suicide, a case Larry and I had discussed a few weeks previously.

There was a certain irony to Blackwell's story. Larry's course was designed to teach physicians how to have open and honest conversations with patients who were asking them to help them die. *No wonder Larry was better at this communication business than I was*, I thought as I read.

I wondered how Larry had answered Blackwell's question about his own death. Blackwell wrote: "Although he [Larry] has no objection to assisted suicide on principle, he said he has decided against it for himself. 'I'm dying and I will die naturally.'"

We didn't meet again until the following Monday, July 22. I'd spent the weekend in thought about an issue that bothered me.

"So the issue that bothers me most is how to deal with the magical thinking that loved ones and caregivers indulge in. How they'll grasp at something, anything, they think might save their loved one. I've observed that in your case too."

"It's a natural reaction to dealing with serious illness in somebody that you love."

"But here's the thing. I find myself doing that same thing now. In the two months we've been meeting, I've got closer to you. I find myself doing that: thinking, if only something could save you."

I was deadly serious of course, but Larry couldn't resist the temptation to tease. "Yeah, will you find something, will you? It's all on your shoulders now." His laugh started deep in his gut and bubbled upwards.

I laughed, but steered him back to the point. This business of hoping for a cure, a miracle, was desperate. I knew it, but I'd still started to indulge in it. Larry offered some reassurance.

"It's part of it. Some of my journal entries just deal with issues in the health-care system, because sometimes that's easier to deal with." I knew what he meant. It's easier to analyze the system than it is to analyze ourselves. It yields more easily to a little scrutiny. Our emotional, spiritual, physical, and psychological states of being, on the other hand, they're more fluid, more difficult to pin down with words. They tend, as the Buddhists say, to resist definition, because the act of definition in some mysterious way diffuses them. They're not concrete, so how can we capture them in concrete words?

He'd been thinking about it too, evidently. For him, he said, it's a question of hope. Cancer patients in particular always hope for a cure. But there comes a point when that's no longer a realistic hope. Larry's been at that point since his diagnosis. So how did he deal with it? Did he just give up, abandon all hope?

"You have to ask yourself, what does hope mean?"

Which sounded utterly cryptic. Surely hope means escaping the crushing weight of dread that the cancer imposes? Hope means cheating it. But for Larry that was not what it meant. For Larry, hope meant finding whatever makes life worth living in your current reality. If a cure is possible, hope for a cure. If your diagnosis is terminal, as his was, refocus your hope. Hope for a calm death, hope your mind remains sharp until the end. Hope your pain is controlled, so your family doesn't have to see you suffer.

"Of course some people can't refocus their hope in this way. They get stuck hoping for a cure irrespective of the situation. In the past, the technique I used to use with those people was to say, Oh yeah, sure, we could have a miracle. Let's say a miracle is possible. But what if there isn't a miracle? How will you support Larry or how will you deal with this particular issue? Some people will never move off of that initial hope, but that's rare. Even my mother-in-law, yesterday she was here, and she came in, and it exhausted me. There was about ten of them here. Putting ten of my relatives in one room is always exhausting, but now my energy levels are so low. So I went to bed and she came to say goodbye. She had tears in her eyes, and she said everything's going to be fine, but her eyes said something different. So I think even she's moved away from that. We haven't told her that I've stopped the chemo and she hasn't asked. I've been very honest with her. I've told her about my cancer and all the rest, but I think with this we just let her down gently. But despite her saying, 'We're going to have a miracle and we have all these people praying for you,' I know the reality. It's trying to balance that that's really difficult for relatives."

"And it's difficult for you too, because you know better than anyone what the reality is."

"Yes, absolutely."

Confront the reality of your situation. Refocus your hope based on that reality. At the most basic level, denial leads to some very bad decisions. It may prevent you from getting your affairs in order. The chaos a terminal diagnosis ushers in can't be tamed by simply sorting out your will, of course, but it can be significantly amplified if you don't attend to these practical matters.

"Do it early," Larry said. "You need to move your little butt and get organized. I know one family, both parents have cancer and they are both having chemo, and they are both dying. But they don't want to talk to their kids about it, so the kids are totally in the dark. Even about what cancer they have and their prognosis. It's destroying their children. They just find it impossible to deal with their parents. Their parents think that they're protecting them, but they have no idea what it's doing. People assume because you can die without a will, that that's okay, but it's not. It means money for a lot of people except your relatives. When you die intestate, it has all sorts of ramifications. You can't do some things and people don't have access to dollars. This couple for example, are relatively well-to-do, and the kids have no access to the money, they have no idea where the money is. They have no idea how to control their parents' business and that's going to lead to really serious problems."

As the disease progresses there will be new challenges to meet. "It's hard for people not going through it to understand, for example, the progressive weakness experienced by cancer patients. And just saying to them, 'Oh, let's get some exercise and go down to the pool, eat a little bit more, you will be stronger, c'mon, you can buck up….' You can't. I can tell you it's very, very frustrating. But it's one of the markers, for me, that my disease is getting worse. Because I have seen it so many times before."

All that can be done, Larry said, is to increase the level of care. "It's all you can do. And it's not just the physical side of things, it's the loss of independence. You become more and more dependent on people. It has psychological and social impacts. It affects the way you interact with people. You can't have hour-long visits. I've watched people as their weakness gets worse. They often become extremely peaceful and less and less interactive with their environment, and that's the way I expect, I hope, that I will go. But it's a matter of preparing your family for that as well. They saw it in me in the first two weeks and it scared the hell out of them. In my drug-addled state they saw I was withdrawing. Nasty business, all of this."

And then there's the loss of appetite, "which is a huge one for families and for the patient as well. If you can't get enough calories in and you're burning them off, you see that candle burning at both ends, and the end is death. But it's not quite that easy and people misunderstand that in particular. It drives families crazy. I know that it's driving Faye crazy. And I just keep telling her I can't. I'm not a kid. You can't force me to eat, I'm not going to eat." It's the question of food again. We've discussed it before, but it's obviously on Larry's mind again.

"She'll put a meal in front of you and then you'll have a few mouthfuls and then…?" I asked.

"No, she actually doesn't do that. She did initially, but now she is much more likely to … especially around suppertime, ask me what I want, what I can tolerate. So we have resolved that. But it took a few weeks. If I left it up to Bella, she would have a plate full of macaroni like this," his hands encircle an imaginary plate of macaroni large enough to feed a small village, "and feed me three times a day."

"That reminds me of my grandmother. She would show her love through food."

"In all families. If you look at … how do we get together and celebrate? Let's go out to dinner. Let's get the family together and have a party. Food is associated with health, it's associated with wealth — it was only the wealthy that could afford to have big parties. It is associated with getting better. If somebody eats more they will get better. It used to be that when the major diseases were infectious diseases, where in the recovery or rehab period, yes, food was important. But it's not as important now when you're dealing with a chronic disease like cancer. More food doesn't result in a longer lifespan."

Which brought us to depression as a symptom. I asked him what we should look for if we suspect someone is depressed. What are the signs?

"It's not just sadness." Larry said. "It's pathological. It means the person exhibits certain symptoms, and sometimes it's really difficult to tell whether they are depressed or if it's their disease or if it's a combination of both. The best person to help you with that is one of your health-care providers. But don't neglect depression. If somebody seems very sad, you need to help that person to deal with it, because when you are in this big, dark hole of depression, you may not see anything except that little patch of sky.

"So they'd look for someone who cries all the time. They'd look for someone who exhibits the sadness and who seems depressed all the time and doesn't smile, and ceases interacting with people around them. They are less engaged in their environment. Things they used to like doing they don't like to do at all now. Not just eating. They don't find any joy in their family … they can't laugh at jokes. There are signs. And often the solution has been medication, but there needs to be more than medication. There needs to be more than a psychiatrist … you need psychosocial support to deal with that…. People need to be aware of it. These are serious symptoms to be aware of … these are symptoms that sometimes get neglected. Pain is something different … pain is common in cancer, and it doesn't have to be feared. You can control a lot of cancer pain. Maybe not all, but you can control a lot of cancer pain. The medications are available for that, but they have side effects, which shouldn't be neglected. But the patient should be encouraged to be as pain-free as possible, because the pain saps their energy and takes away from their ability to deal with the things that they have to deal with. It takes away their quality of life."

We finished up a little early, because Larry had practical financial issues of his own to deal with. His financial consultant was calling at eleven o'clock to discuss financial vehicles for his estate. "She called me and wanted to set this up. I think I know more about the legal and financial stuff than many of these consultants. They know all about the actual physical structure of things like trusts and companies and corporations, and of course they want to protect my insurance money. But it is protected, because it's tax-free. My financial consultant thought there was another vehicle that we could use. So ... my accountant and this financial consultant and somebody else from her office set up an appointment for me to go there today. They did this five weeks ago. I said, 'And you expect me to be there, do you?' It caught her off-guard. I said, 'Well, you know, I may have to cancel. I may not be able to go in. You may have to come here.' Then I said to her, 'Are the things that you are thinking of going to take more than a month or two?'

"'Oh yeah,' she said, 'they may take three, four, five months.'

"So I told her I shouldn't even embark on them. I ain't going to be around to sign the final papers. So we will see what they have to say. She's really been taken aback by my illness in total and how weak I am. The whole idea is about making money for themselves and for others, and my idea is to protect whatever assets I have. But mixed in there is this terrible illness. You're asking someone to make decisions on important questions, but how do you know the person has good decision-making capacity when Librach's way off on the medication? How do you assess that?"

It's a fair point, although since giving up the chemo Larry's usual mental acuity seemed to have returned. There was certainly nothing wrong with his memory. In his case I didn't think it would be a problem, but it's easy to see how vulnerable a patient confused by chemo brain could be to the unscrupulous. Which bolsters the argument to get the financial business taken care of early.

"So we'll see what happens at 11:00. They are going to call. I said I can't go in to see them. I can't go down there and have an hour-and-a-half meeting there and an hour and a half of going back and forth. It's a hot, humid day. I ain't going nowhere."

CHAPTER 21

alive

My father sported the same haircut his entire life: the regulation cut mandated by the Royal Marines when he enlisted. He was a small-c conservative in an age of rapid change, a conformist in an era of individualism. The tide of change that swept through England in the mid-sixties confused and isolated him, made him feel like an outsider, an alien, but it didn't faze my eldest brother. Not only did John embrace it, he seemed to me to shape it.

At eighteen, and a full-grown man to my eyes, he returned home from a six-month trip to the Far East. It must have been a weekend, because I was home and irrepressibly excited. My mother had banished me to my bedroom to await his arrival. Fortunately my room was at the front of the house, so I hoisted open the sash window and swung myself out; far enough to see the bottom of the road if I stretched my neck. To a ten-year-old the wait felt interminable, but I was finally rewarded by an outlandish vision. A tall man turned the corner, his hair bleached blond by the sun, corkscrew curled by the sea, his face and arms the colour of a chestnut. He looked like some exotic bird in our dull little street. The transformation was so unexpected and complete I wasn't sure it was my brother until he was a few houses away, at which point I leant further out of the window and started to wave and call out to him.

He hadn't cut his hair in the six months since he left. It was longer and more outrageous-looking than the hairstyles of any of the era's pop stars:

the Rolling Stones and the Beatles included. When he reached the front door he rang the doorbell, and we exchanged greetings while he waited for someone to open it. That person was my father, who refused to let him into the house until he'd had "a decent hair cut."

Even shorn of his golden curls, John stood out, with his necklaces, bracelets, his tie-dyed Ts or paisley-patterned shirts. One day I arrived home to find a pair of Levi's crumpled in four inches of water at the bottom of the bathtub. The odour of household bleach hung in the air. "Don't touch those, kiddo" he told me. I asked what he was doing but he refused to explain. Tapping his forefinger on the side of his nose to indicate I should keep mine out of business that didn't concern me, he said: "Just wait and you'll see, won't you?"

When they emerged from the bath the following day they were mottled like Friesian cattle. But John still wasn't satisfied. While he sat watching the TV that night he patiently unpicked the hem and the outside seam to the knee, frayed the bottom inch or so of the jeans and stitched brightly coloured cotton panels into each leg. When he was finished he looked, according to my father, "idiotic, like a scarecrow, or a lunatic."

I don't suppose my father realized that the English word *idiot* is derived from the same root Greek word as *idiosyncratic.*

I didn't quite know what to make of it all. Within a couple of years this style of clothing would be commonplace in London, but at that time John was a spot of bright colour in a sea of greys and indigos. He certainly attracted attention whenever he walked along the street. Heads turned, children pointed, old men shook their heads, and old women tutted audibly as we passed.

I found the attention alarming. Like most ten-year-old boys, I spent most of my time trying to evade the notice of adults, so for John to court outrage challenged my world view.

Like the books I devoured as a child, John opened my eyes to other worlds, other possibilities, to the truth that we can shape ourselves according to our own tastes. I realized I didn't have to allow others to define and constrain my choices because he demonstrated the truth of it for me.

And while it's true that, at ten, I idealized my oldest brother and probably encouraged his tendency to embellish his seaman's tales, it's also undeniable that he was the first to teach me that exciting and exotic worlds could be reached by opening my front door, as well as by opening the cover of a book. That such worlds were not just imaginary. They were real, and one day I could reach them.

Stephen drove to Oldham without stopping. He arrived just after two o'clock in the afternoon.

We don't see the dying often enough to recognize the signs, but a palliative-care physician becomes familiar with them: the patient's breath slows and there may be long gaps between breaths. The patient may stop blinking, and as the blood circulation slows certain changes in their skin will be noticeable: it may become blue or blotchy, the mouth may turn bluish grey, the face may become pale, the fingertips may darken, and the nose, ears, feet, arms, and legs may feel cool to the touch. Also, the skin on the underside of the body may darken.

Stephen parked the car and ran to John's room. Shirley sat at John's bedside. Her eight-year-old daughter, Ki'anna, stood at the foot of the bed. "John was laid prone, but he was breathing," Stephen said. "Shirley greeted me. She gripped John's hand as if she were trying her best to stop him leaving."

He took John's hand and was surprised to feel John's grip tighten around his.

It can sometimes happen. An unresponsive patient can suddenly become alert, experience a sudden surge of energy. They may even become talkative, and report being hungry or interested in seeing visitors. It's short lived.

In John's case it was no more than the sudden tightening of his grip around his brother's hand. Seconds later Stephen heard a rattle from his throat.

I've never heard the so-called death rattle, but it understandably frightens many caregivers who are at the side of their dying loved ones. It has a simple physical explanation: it's caused by a build-up of saliva and phlegm in the back of the throat. The patient isn't conscious enough to cough and clear the buildup. But although it's disturbing to hear, it's not dangerous. It won't choke the patient, and it's not uncomfortable for them. If they're not conscious enough to cough, they're not conscious enough to feel it. People sometimes ask if a suction pump can be used to clear it, but that can cause the patient to gag or vomit, which definitely will distress them. Sometimes palliative-care physicians will prescribe drugs to manage this symptom.

In John's case this rattle accompanied his last breath. "I could tell he'd stopped breathing. It was no more than thirty seconds after I arrived," Stephen said.

That's not always the case. In some cases the rattling, gurgling breathing can go on for hours or even a few days. It may be accompanied by a change in breathing patterns. The patient's breath may speed up, sound shallow, or become irregular. But just before death the breathing slows down. There may be as long as twenty or thirty seconds between breaths, and the patient may sound as if they're gasping. Again, this is distressing to witness, but the patient won't be experiencing distress. They won't even be aware of the change.

Stephen went to find one of the home's staff. The staff member ushered the three of them out of the room and checked John's breathing. He confirmed John was dead. "We had to hang around the home for a while to get the death certificate and other paperwork, so arrangements could be made," Stephen said. Numbed as he was by John's death, he felt hurried into decisions. It seemed to him the home was in a hurry to get the body out of the room, and a new resident in. It seemed "unseemly."

If John had been cared for by Larry or one of his colleagues, there's no doubt in my mind his death would have been handled with more compassion, and a greater understanding that the grieving are just as worthy of care and attention as the dying.

Whenever I've told Canadian palliative-care physicians how badly my brother's case was handled, I'm uniformly met with incredulity. The U.K. is supposed to be the gold standard of end-of-life care. It was developed there, and has been an integral part of the health-care system for longer than any other country. I simply shrug my shoulders and point out that even the best systems sometimes fail.

I come back to the question I've asked myself since John died. What difference would it have made if his care had been handled better? John would still have died. His family and loved ones would still have grieved. Would anything have been any different?

I found one answer to this question unexpectedly, when I asked Stephen for his account of John's death. I originally asked him in February 2015. It took him almost five months to respond. Not because he was lazy, too busy, or wasn't interested. It took five months because it stirred up difficult memories and made him question his role in John's death. He wondered if he'd done everything he could have done for our brother, if he'd made enough of an effort to comfort him as he was dying, if he'd really understood what John needed.

Stephen's struggle to respond to my request is another symptom of the poor care John received, because, as Larry used to say, palliative care treats the family as well as the dying patient. And by family he meant all of the loved ones of the dying person, whether or not they were related by blood ties.

In truth, there was probably little or nothing Stephen could have done any differently to help John, but Stephen's outcome would have been so much better if he'd been allowed to air his questions years ago, and had received the assurance of a professional that he'd done all he could.

In his later years, fashion trends caught up with and rapidly overtook John. The outlandish alien I remembered from my childhood was completely gone by the time he reached his forties. But he remained an iconoclast and a nonconformist. When he first realized he was dying, he chose the music he wanted at his funeral: Frankie Goes to Hollywood's "Relax." He had no control over the choice of officiant at his funeral. We, his siblings, had little to no choice either, and circumstances conspired to give us perhaps the last vicar in all of Oldham that John would have chosen. He was, to our lax twenty-first-century minds, at the extreme end of the traditionalist spectrum, and would brook no deviation from the traditional funeral service, limiting us to one (very brief) eulogy. But John won a small point. He would have savoured the look of intense discomfort on the vicar's face, when Frankie's throbbing, sexual beat filled the tiny chapel at the crematorium as his coffin was brought in. He would even have appreciated the look of relief that washed over the man's face when whoever was in charge of the audio cut the lyric before the words "when you wanna come." I can't swear to it that everyone in the place smiled, but most of the people I could see were either openly smiling or trying to hide a grin behind their hand.

In this regard at least, he managed to preserve something of himself at his funeral. In most other respects the essential components of my brother were long gone by the time his physical body expired.

If one component of a good death is dying as you have lived, John died badly. The cancer and the institution stripped away his persona, his bright-burning character, and left a husk. Not having known him before the cancer, the doctors, nurses, and caregivers couldn't see beyond his emaciated frame to the spirit of the man within it.

John's physical body died on July 14, 2010, but he died weeks before that. So I return to the question I asked myself the last time I saw him: what was the point of keeping that spent husk alive in those final few weeks? His life was not dignified and honoured in his dying. In fact, everything about those last few weeks dishonoured my memories of him, because he was forced, at last, to conform to the requirements of the system, to die as they demanded.

CHAPTER 22

Narrative

I've hated exclamation marks for as long as I can remember. There's a reason newspaper sub-editors call them screamers. They're the loud guy in the meeting who speaks over everyone else, the overdressed woman at the party, the kid throwing a tantrum in the supermarket. The exclamation mark is the bratty member of the punctuation family. And yet Larry's final words as I packed my bag at the end of our meeting on July 22 almost merited one. Certainly they made my pulse quicken.

"I think I may have eight weeks left where I'm strong enough to work."

Eight weeks. He wondered if it was going to be long enough.

"It will have to be," I said.

On July 26, I called Larry to find out what had happened at his CT scan the previous day. The tumour had grown. The chemo hadn't halted its progression. It may have slowed it down, but not by much.

What did that mean? Nothing more than we already knew. Modern instruments (CT scans, MRIs, X-rays) open us up, reveal what would once have been hidden. In another age the tumour would have progressed in silence, eating him from the inside out, with nobody the wiser.

But our instruments, wondrous though they are, will still be judged by generations to come as crude and ineffective. What use is it to measure the progress of a known fatal condition? It is watching a tragedy unfold that we have no power to prevent. How much better if our instruments were sensitive enough to detect the first cancerous cluster of cells before they explode into a full-blown tumour?

A bad habit of mine, this; I could inoculate myself from the pain of this news if I analyzed and intellectualized. Analysts call it deflection.

It was clear the last spark of hope had died. It was in Faye's tired and stretched voice when I spoke with her. It was in Larry's. He wanted, I think, to talk about how this felt for him. He reached out to me over the telephone. He sounded vulnerable and afraid, for the first time. I changed the subject. I spoke of this or that practical issue to do with our work. When I put the phone down I was a little disgusted with myself. I felt I had let him down, that I'd flinched.

I knew (I told myself) he needed these meetings, our conversations, now — they helped him create the narrative he had chosen to craft. And that's the reality of all human lives when it comes down to it, isn't it? That we choose the narrative we write with our lives every day. By the decisions we make, by the ways we choose to spend our days, we craft the lives we live in, our story. You might say this is bullshit. That our lives are easily thrown off course by luck or circumstance. A tornado, a tsunami, a global financial crisis. Who can resist those forces? And you'd be right. Many things, perhaps most things, are totally beyond our control.

But that doesn't absolve us. Consider Larry. His cancer was as devastating as a tsunami. If he'd had any choice in the matter I'm sure he would have refused the chance to experience cancer. But that's not the point. It wasn't the cancer that crafted Larry's narrative, but the choices he made after he knew about it. Larry chose to die, as he had lived, with purpose. It was only that, only his intent, that gave his death meaning. But it was enough. More than enough.

The following Monday, July 29, I was supposed to visit Larry for another session. I planned to bring up the subject of physician-assisted death again. It had been on my mind a lot as I saw him slipping away, as a little bit more of Larry was extinguished with every visit. I thought back to John. In those last days and hours, what was the point of keeping him alive? Some small part of me had wanted to smother him with his pillow rather than watch him suffer. But it would have taken the kind of courage I perhaps don't have.

I thought I'd bring up the *National Post* story Larry was quoted in. The online version of that story had attracted a long discussion string. Most comments came from the family or loved ones of someone who had been kept alive beyond what they felt was necessary or humane. The commentators saw the problem from the patient's point of view, ignoring the doctor's dilemma. But of course a physician is put in a horrible position as the person who would administer this so-called peaceful, gentle death. Everywhere it's legal there are safeguards in place, but even so, killing people is not why they became doctors.

I called as usual at around 8:50, and spoke to Faye. She said Larry had had a bad weekend and that David Kendal was visiting that morning, which was a bad sign. When I had arranged the meeting on Thursday, Larry wasn't scheduled to see David.

I promised to call back later in the day. Around 11:45 I got an email from Larry, asking me to call him. I didn't see it for ten minutes. When I did I called straight away. He sounded not-quite Larry on the phone. His voice a half tone lower, the humour knocked out of it.

He said he was feeling weaker every day, wanted to meet as soon as possible. I offered to go over in the afternoon, but he said his family was visiting to discuss the arrangements for his care. Another bad sign. I arranged to visit the first thing the following morning.

Later that afternoon there was a flurry of phone calls between CTV, Faye, and me. The station's *W5* documentary team had been working on a story about Larry's death for several weeks. (Larry had trained CTV's Dr. Marla Shapiro earlier in her career.) Though they'd already got some interviews with Faye and Larry in the can, there were a few follow-up questions they wanted to ask.

Wanting to protect Faye and his family, Larry suggested they film us working together. The plan was to film on Thursday, August 8. Meanwhile, the previous Friday (July 26) Larry had been informed that Mount Sinai Hospital (MSH) had planned a reception for him on Tuesday, August 6. CTV planned to film both the MSH reception and Larry and me while we worked on the book.

But things quickly changed. Larry called MSH to cancel his participation in the reception in his honour, and Faye emailed the CTV team to tell them Larry wouldn't be attending. She mentioned he wasn't at all well, and had really deteriorated in the past week.

That was the email that provoked the flurry of activity from the CTV team as they scrambled to get their second interview while they still could.

CTV's Steve Bandera called me to coordinate. It was okay with me if it was okay with Faye and Larry. They agreed. It was a go.

The condo was a hive when I turned up, a little before 9:30. It wasn't so much the extra bodies — there were just three members of the CTV crew after all, Steve, Bill, and Anton — but the extra energy. Things were usually tranquil at Larry's, well ordered. Life moved at a different pace. I noticed the bustle as I removed my shoes and entered the living room, the sheer industry of it all: tables and chairs moved, cables taped to the hardwood floor, equipment everywhere, and a barrage of calls to and from the CTV offices, voices raised where voices were normally measured and gentle.

I was the last to arrive, but they were still setting up. Faye told me Larry was in the bedroom. "He's very tired," she said. "He probably won't be able to give them more than about fifteen minutes."

The second I saw him I knew she was right. He was fully dressed, in a striped short-sleeved button-down and a pair of khaki trousers. But he lay flat on the bed, his hands folded across his chest, the curtains drawn against the bright sunlight outside.

"How do you feel?"

He moved his head slightly, but barely stirred. "Tired. I don't think I'll have the energy to give them much. It'll be up to you I'm afraid."

"I'll tell them to go easy on you. You have to let them know when you've had enough."

Back in the living room I let Anton (the executive producer and the man who would interview Larry) know that he didn't feel well, that if he called a halt to things they'd have to stop.

They wanted a shot of us working together, what TV people call B-roll material, to run in the background during voiceover. Even so, the shot had to be carefully set up and it all took time. Finally they were ready for us, and Larry somehow gathered enough strength to stand. He was using a walker by this time, so I helped him up off the bed, moved the walker to within grabbing distance, and we made slow progress into his study, where the camera had been set up. To the TV crew it was a minimally invasive kit: one camera and a mike boom. Nothing over the top. To an invalid using a walker it looked like a particularly challenging assault course, what with the trip wires (the cabling) and the hurdles (the tripod). We helped him navigate through the hazards. "You trying to make sure I don't make a fast getaway?" Larry alluded to *W5*'s reputation for confrontational reporting. There was polite laughter and some further banter back and forth, but I could feel their relief ripple around the room: he had enough energy to crack a joke.

They needed us both in shot. Normally we sat across from each other, the mike between. A comfortable divide. That wouldn't work here. I grabbed Larry's footstool and dragged it next to his chair. "This okay?" I got the thumbs up, but it felt a little odd, to be this close to my "subject." An unaccustomed intimacy.

They set us both up with mikes, but it was a false start. Somebody's mike didn't work. They were both retrieved, the batteries changed (Bill seemed to have an inexhaustible store of them), and we tried again. This time it was successful, but there was another delay as the CTV crew went into the living room to discuss some technical aspect of the shot. While we waited Larry said, "When we last did this I was wearing a shirt that fit not too badly. I put that same shirt on today and the arms were down here." He indicated a point on his upper arm about halfway down his bicep. The first *W5* interview had been little over three weeks before.

The CTV crew trooped back into the room and we started our usual chat as if they were not there.

"How have you felt this week?"

"Much worse. It's very surprising, although not surprising from the point of view of knowing where I was heading. And it's not depression. It's a couple of things. A complete lack of strength. I feel like I can't get out of bed every morning. It's crazy. During the night I wake up and I'm able to get up and go to the washroom. But all of a sudden in the morning I don't want to get out of bed. It's really … it's incredible weakness. And also what I am sensing is a withdrawal from things around me. My family talked about this yesterday. We had a family conference to talk about this … is that sense of, I need to push back, I've done what I can. I find the energy levels are not there, and people don't understand that, they really don't. Patients have described it to me, but were never really able to describe it perfectly. And I don't think that I could describe it now. It's like somebody has opened a stopcock in the bottom of your tank, and just left it open and you just don't … you put anything in the top and it comes out the bottom right away."

It struck me like a blow. It had been over a week since we last recorded an interview. Then his speech had been quite clear. But now he was slurring. I listened carefully as he answered my question; the decline was quite marked, he was sliding over words, mashing them slightly.

"And that extends even to breathing?"

"Yes, I guess I'm having difficulty breathing. I don't feel like I have any energy to take the next breath and taking that next breath takes a lot of energy and thinking. The other thing that is happening is my cognitive abilities … it's like my life is in snippets of things. Partly TV, partly what happened last week, partly what is happening now. Even my dreams are in snippets of things. Not really a cohesive sort of dream or fantasy, or whatever you want to call it. I'm forgetting simple things. It worries me. Can I put it together in a way that people will understand what that means, because I have seen it so often in patients? Now that I am experiencing it, there's one hell of a difference."

He believed it's a normal part of the process of dying, but the oncologists he'd mentioned it to were skeptical. They regarded it as a myth. Why, I wondered? "Maybe it's because the care for dying patients is increasingly being passed off to palliative physicians. Maybe the oncologists really don't get to see patients at this stage of disease progression."

"And what do you think is causing your cognitive decline? Maybe the tumour is invading your brain or…?"

"No, I don't think it's a brain tumour. You see this often enough with all cancers. Especially as you enter that final phase. I'm worried about my brain, sure … but I'm lucky in that I've got one of the cancer groups that doesn't metastasize to the brain very easily. I'm not worried about that as much as: how much will I be able to continue on and be of value to me and my family? That was one of the things that we talked about last night at our family conference. It's the first time that Faye and I and the kids have had a chance to sit down alone and speak about these things. Telling them that if I seem withdrawn, I am withdrawing. It's not their fault. If it seems I'm not able to quite have it there, yes, they're right. It's frightening for them."

"Yes, because you have always been so present."

"Yes, very present to them. Lacking that presence is something they feel acutely. I've … in our family care plan, I'm really handing over now a lot of the stuff to them. At a time when Faye is already feeling incredible pressure."

"What was the conclusion of that discussion?"

"They are going to need to ramp up and they have each taken on some of the responsibility for certain things. I need to speak to certain family members because I can't do visitors like I could do before. Even a half hour for a visitor to me is interminable. There's nothing wrong with my visitors, it's me that is the problem.

"So that is going to be an issue ... reducing phone calls —" In a moment of unrehearsable irony, Larry's phone rang as these words left his lips. We couldn't help but laugh at it, but Larry got us back on track almost immediately: "... giving them certain responsibilities around the phone calls and we developed a tier system ... people just don't realize that I can't ... it takes energy to speak and breathe. It takes energy to cope with the stuff that is going through your mind because now my prognosis is definitely down to weeks or ... it's really not down to a long time. I mean, I've had my time. It's been four months since my diagnosis and the beginnings of treatment. Have I savoured every moment? No, I've had my tough times, but it's really a pleasure to have had the time that I had to be able to do what I did and to get the kids' memory boxes done, to settle things with my family. You never quite finish all of your tasks. There will be things I'm not going to finish and giving up on those was a big step for me."

Larry wasn't telling his friends and family not to visit, just that they didn't have to sit at his bedside holding his hand. They were welcome to come by and sit out in the living room. He didn't, he said, need his hand held. "That's not what we need. At this stage we need support. One of the things that I have learned through palliative care is that you don't have to do things to people. You just have to be there for them. And I know it sounds trite, but often it's just a matter of them knowing that you are there ... is the most important thing...."

It was a critical step for Larry. He'd always been such a social person, and had enjoyed having his friends and extended family around him. That he now found this too much to cope with was a significant admission. He must have agonized over this decision.

There was another worry on his mind too. It seemed clearer than ever that he wouldn't be around when the book was written, and he was worried about who would stand in for him, fact check the manuscript, make sure it didn't do any harm. "I don't want to do people harm, but on the other hand I don't want to sugar-coat everything. It may be that you are going to have to proceed with a proxy from me now. In two weeks I may not be able to speak. It's frightening."

Anton interrupted us. They had their ten minutes of tape. They were going to move the equipment to the lounge: there were a few more questions they wanted to ask Larry, and they wanted to interview me. Larry and I continued our interview while they set up.

Perhaps it was the sudden silence in the room, or the unaccustomed intimacy of sitting at Larry's left hand; perhaps what he had just told me about the decision to limit visits, or the slurring in his speech. I don't know. But something struck me to the core. I was frozen, drowning in a grief that was both sudden and utterly unexpected. My patina of professionalism completely stripped away. I felt naked and raw.

I'll never know if Larry carried on talking out of politeness, or if he simply didn't notice that I was frozen, but for the next few minutes he continued to talk, skipping, Larry-like, from topic to topic. Finally my tongue loosened.

"This is hard, isn't it?" It was all I could find to say.

"Holy shit, it is. But you can't ignore the invitation to die. People go all throughout life saying, but why is this happening to me? Well, you were born. After that everything else is going to happen to you."

He paused. We both did. He looked down at his hands. The shaking from his Parkinson's seemed to be worse this morning too. "Cancelling the event next week had a lot of ripples in it. I'm surprised how many people have reacted."

He looked up, away from his mutinous hands. "My hands are so shaky. If I'd taken my medication this morning it would have been helpful...."

"Do you want me to get it for you?" And just like that I'd crossed the wafer-thin line to caregiver. It was a small thing, to be sure, to run to his bathroom cabinet to find and fetch his medication, and perhaps I'm freighting it with unnecessary significance. It was something anyone would have done, even a child. Larry's granddaughters would, no doubt, have thought nothing of fetching Zaide's pills. I know this. Yet with this small act of service, so commonly given (and received, on behalf of the cared for), I had gone from observer to participant.

Anton's silhouette appeared in the doorframe. They were ready for us. Larry navigated his walker to the chair they'd placed in the middle of the sitting room. I wasn't needed yet, so I sat on the couch and watched. The camera, sound, everything was good. They were ready to go.

I watched Larry inflate. From somewhere, deep down inside him, he drew on a reserve of energy. The tiredness left his voice, he sat visibly straighter in his chair, and the slur in his speech had almost disappeared.

Anton had his questions prepared and cycled through them. Larry was sharp and he knew his subject. He had become an expert at covering up the physical impacts of his cancer. Aside from his chemo hair, most people wouldn't have seen any evidence of decline. But I'd spent the past three months with him. He was doing a great job, but it was obvious his mental acuity was dulling a little. I could spot the cracks that may not have been evident to Anton and his crew: the slight hesitancy over word choice, the few small slips he made, and the rapid flow of information, usually so effortless, wasn't there for him today. Also, there was an increase in Larry's vocal tics. He had a number of them he used to fill in gaps in the conversation. "And all the rest" was his favourite, and it was present with a new abundance during the interview.

It was interesting that Larry himself described his symptoms (the fragmented dreams and even his increasingly fragmented reality) as "interesting." It was an odd word choice, but understandable. He was still analyzing, still trying to preserve his distant scientific perspective, even as he suffered. That must be what it takes to be a physician: the ability to achieve that remove.

They filmed for half an hour or more, which surprised me. I thought he would call a halt fifteen minutes in; he'd seemed so exhausted when I'd first arrived at the condo, but Larry seemed to hold up to it well.

But when it was over he headed straight for his bedroom while they miked me for my interview. While we prepared, Anton and I chatted about his interview with Larry. He mentioned how hard he found it to be direct about death. He'd used euphemisms for death when he was questioning Larry. He couldn't be direct, couldn't say: "When you die." I sympathized. I'd stumbled a couple of times myself. Even though Larry had always talked openly about dying and death, and it was easier to talk to him directly about his own death than it would have been with anyone else, the social norms are powerful around this subject. It's not quite as bad as taking out your genitalia in public, but it's close. That's why we resort to euphemism. That's how powerful our cultural denial of death is. We find it next to impossible to overcome our social mores.

Halfway into my interview the doorbell went. It was Larry's nurse. When we finished up our interview Anton wondered aloud if this would be a good opportunity to get some footage of home-based care in action. He was focused on telling his story in the most powerful way possible, of course. As was I. "Well," I said, "I think Larry's pretty tired, but you can ask him." While I removed the mike and gathered my own things together, Anton was petitioning for a last favour from Larry. I was surprised when he agreed, "as long as it's OK with the nurse." I left them setting up the equipment again, this time in Larry's bedroom.

Later that week Larry emailed his circle of friends and confidants what he called his "Penultimate update":

> Things are changing rapidly for me. I am getting weaker day by day. My brain seems to be working much more sporadically now making it difficult to hold conversations and making it more difficult to finish my book (almost there though!).
>
> I appreciate all your warm wishes. We are going to limit my visitors so have patience with us. We will not be able to accommodate all your requests but please keep emails and notes coming as they will be answered by me and/or family members. They are important to us.
>
> It has been quite a ride and as I approach the end of my journey, I want to thank you all for your friendship, support and love over the years.

CHAPTER 23

Cure

Larry was sprawled over his crumpled sheets, little black devices (the TV remote, the remote that operated the bed, the cordless handset) scattered around him on the bed, like the exoskeletons of a family of mutant insects, like so many discarded ideas. He was sweating heavily. Not that he was mopping his brow or even that he was slick with perspiration, but there was a towel laid over his pillow and he was wearing only boxers and what appeared to be a soccer shirt. Natalie, who was with me, told me later it reminded her of her father during his last few weeks: the clothing, the swollen belly, the wasted limbs, the chemo fuzz that was all that was left of his hair. And his face, shrunken and slightly wizened, the well-groomed moustache the one feature untouched by the disease. But of course I thought of John the last time I saw him.

These echoes are impossible to suppress. We're pattern-seeking creatures, we humans. We make these connections to short-circuit the process of analysis and evaluation. We use comparisons like yardsticks, rules of thumb to help us draw faster conclusions.

Impossible too not to do a mental assessment of Larry's condition. Where were we now? How far from death? A week? Two?

It was Monday, August 5, another low-energy day, though he seemed in good spirits. But judging from the way he continually reached for his sippy cup, he was parched. And he slurred his words more noticeably. But he still seemed relatively alert mentally, still with us. Every time I saw him, though, there was a fractional loss of cognitive function. As if he were escaping a little every day, like helium from a balloon. I could see him hunt down the right word as he talked, halting to wait for the path to reveal itself, scenting it out, and sometimes failing.

He'd always been so sharp, had always chosen the exact word he wanted, so this was painful to see, the worst aspect of the disease. Larry *was* his mental acuity. He was defined by the speed of his wit, his access to a vast pool of stored knowledge — was inseparable from it. It would be easy to overdramatize these moments. To pretend they were bigger than they were. The truth is they were easy to miss unless I was paying attention. I suspect most of the time Larry would have liked to have covered them up, although he was frank enough about them if I came straight out and asked, or if I came at them from an angle: the lack of understanding of this slipping away, the lack of research, the lack even of interest in the phenomenon. It was easier to talk about these things in an abstract way.

But it frustrated him, particularly the progressive weakness he experienced. He'd often heard about it from his patients, but now he was experiencing it first-hand and he said it was "annoying, demoralizing, and intractable. It really is hard to describe. There's a definite physical component to it. It's difficult to get out of the chair, take a shower, or walk around the condo. But there's also an emotional component. It impacts my independence and makes me more reliant on others. Makes me feel more of a burden."

He shared with me the notes he wrote on the topic in his journal:

> It's now 8 a.m. I've been asleep since nine o'clock last evening. I was used to getting up at 6 a.m. every morning. Now that I have the luxury of being able to sleep in later you'd think I'd be happy. I'm not. Even though I have an easy sleep most nights, when I wake up I don't feel refreshed. In fact I often lie there for several minutes wondering how I'll push myself out of bed. I'm finally able to get out of bed but I need to walk very slowly, hanging on to walls and dressers. I drag myself into the kitchen to get a glass of juice then return to my nice comfortable bed. It seems to me that someone has drained all my energy from my body. But I push myself and manage to get dressed although that leads to the need to take another period of rest.

> My family look at me and think I can do more. Everyone who visits says I look very good. If only they could feel what I feel — that every movement and almost every breath must be taken with some effort. They exhort me — exercise more, eat more, don't give in. But I really don't have energy to even think about doing any of those things. It's overwhelming, a pernicious symptom that often lacks external signs except for general wasting when that is present.

"You said something interesting last week about oncologists not recognizing this weakness and loss of cognitive function because they've very often given over care of their patients to palliative-care physicians by the time it happens. Have you thought any more about that? That seems to me something that oncologists need to hear."

"I think they do need to hear it. They need to hear it from the horse's mouth. But they've also got to be open to hearing it. They've got to be able to … they always look to do diagnosis. If they could do a CT scan of the cognitive functions that would be great, but they need to know what they're looking for, and they need to spend more time with people. But they're not going to do that at the end of life…. If you speak to people like Gary Rodin at Princess Margaret Hospital, who has a psychosocial oncology and palliative-care program, he sees this a lot. But trying to get referrals for people or trying to get oncologists to understand this is really very difficult. It either gets blamed on the chemo or it gets blamed on the disease or it gets blamed on the palliative-care docs: 'they don't know what they're talking about,' and maybe we don't, but I haven't seen much in the literature in the past about this. But I've seen that withdrawal, I've seen those changes. I've seen the memory that gets poorer: does it have a nutritional component to it? I mean there are many things left to study in this area."

"Presumably the tumour is affecting all sorts of chemical processes in the body? Would you theorize it's a hormonal or chemical imbalance?"

"With cancer, yes. I mean it's both a reaction of the body against the tumour and the reaction and interplay of tumours with the body, so there's both. And it's more common with certain cancers, particularly lung and pancreatic cancer, but also leukemias and lymphomas.

You're seeing chemicals produced by both. So do they have cognitive impact? Probably, but there hasn't been a lot of study. So whether it's reversible or not, whether you're actually losing neurons or … nobody does functional MRI scanning with people like this … or if they have they certainly haven't entered the literature that I've seen, or entered the mainstream oncology literature."

He shifted, twisted on the bed, tried to get more comfortable, to unstick himself from the sheets, but he hadn't lost his train of thought. "So you'd think there'd be interest, but there's no interest. The interest in cancer is cure. That's where the money is, that's where the dollars are and all of cancer is, you know, it's … pharmaceutical companies. They're the ones that have the money. To bring a new drug to market is what? A billion, two billion dollars now? And they're not interested in studying anything that doesn't cure cancer or prolong life. They certainly don't see it as their research priority, or their pipeline of drugs or whatever."

"But when you're thinking about quality of life at the end of life, keeping someone's cognitive function going as long as possible is one of the critical elements, you would have thought?"

"That's to you and me." Larry lifted his hand to his face, pantomime style, and stage whispered to Natalie, "We've brainwashed him. He didn't see that little thing by his pillow at night.

"Yeah, no, you need to see it and then you need to have the strength to figure out how you might want to study it. I'm not a researcher. Never was, never will be a researcher." He stopped himself again. One of those moments when death's invisible presence in the room asserted itself. "Especially now. But those are interesting questions and those are the things that people need to pick up on. But the current cancer research piece all the money goes to PMH or the Cancer Society. They're more interested in patient care than they ever were, but mostly around chemotherapy and cure. The money that's available beyond cancer treatment or research is very limited."

"Isn't there anything that can be done, anything the patient can do to slow it down or stave it off?"

"Well, there's some evidence that mild exercise, especially early on, can make a difference later. You might be able to delay the onset of weakness, and its severity as it develops."

Larry had made a list in his journal — of course he had — of measures to help patients who are very weak.

> Most importantly, we have to educate the patient, family and health-care providers about the causes and approaches to this symptom. Then there's the exercise, not only to maintain strength but also balance. You could try different approaches: exercise bikes, walks outdoors or in safe indoor environments and gentle swimming exercises. Physiotherapists and occupational therapists can also help with this. At some stage though you're going to have to resort to canes, walkers, wheelchairs and other mobility aids. Again, it's important the patient and their family are instructed on how to use them effectively. If they're not educated properly, and they're not using them properly, they won't see the benefit and will probably stop using them. And, as the weakness progresses and the patient has to spend more time in bed or in chairs you need to pay more attention to skincare. Adjustable beds like hospital beds and chairs that provide effective support are helpful.

But what about his own decline? I couldn't tell if he was just frustrated that nobody would listen to him or affronted by their failure to accept his self-prognosis. "I feel things slipping quickly. I'd love to be proved wrong, but even Russell seems to have this attitude that I'm doing much better than I think I am."

Nobody else was taking him seriously, he said, because he looked okay, "except for the bumps where I used to have tissue mass. But I'm not exaggerating things. I can feel it. But it's really hard to convince people that you might be a few weeks away from death when you seem to be doing okay."

What he failed to account for is our natural propensity to think wishfully. Interesting that even seasoned professionals find themselves prone to this when they're emotionally attached to the patient. They only wanted to give him longer. They saw all the hopeful signs and were wilfully ignorant (it seemed) about the negative ones. And here was Larry insisting, "Damnit, I'm dying, I tell you. Why won't you people believe me?"

It was a new danger, this weakness. It put him at new risks. "I had a fall the other day, in the bathroom. I fell backwards. I didn't really hit my head. I fell onto the toilet of all things, and my head went back. But I never lost consciousness.

"Albert happened to call me about fifteen minutes later, to ask how I was doing. I told him I was very tired, first thing in the morning I'm very tired, I can barely think about breathing, never mind anything else. He said, 'You're slurring your words.' I said, 'I know I'm just very tired and my mouth is dry, let me take some water.' He said, 'No, I'm coming over right away.' So he came over to find this weak old fart not being able to … you know, I was fine. I said, 'I could have told you that, Albert. I didn't lose consciousness. My brain is as bad as it's always been. Just leave me alone.'"

Larry stopped to consider and obviously decided he'd been a little hard on Albert, because he felt the need to elaborate: "But he's good otherwise. There was that sudden change last week that sort of set things off, and he was good with my family and he's really … he really helped Faye and the kids understand what's going on. So that was good. He's amazing with his patients."

I'd been avoiding it, because I knew it was a painful topic for Larry, but I couldn't avoid the question of how his family had reacted to the decision he made last week to limit visits.

"Still too many people want to visit. People don't seem to understand the pressure. It really is very, very difficult to say no to people, it's also difficult to say yes … yesterday my mother-in-law wanted to come down. Well, she can come down only if somebody brings her. That means my sister-in-law and my brother-in-law. Well my nephew is in town for a year's" — he stopped, corrected himself — "month's sabbatical" — he paused again, hunted the right word, breathed out in exasperation, before he found it — "program at Toronto Western here. So he came with his wife. Then Judith came with Ryan, you know, and so it turned out … Faye was just beside herself.

"She's the one I'm worried about now. We had a long talk last night about it. People don't seem to understand. It's nothing personal, it's just we don't have the energy."

It frustrated him that he had to repeat the same story for each visitor. The same questions, with every new visitor: How is he feeling? Is he well?

"I just want to record it, or put a flag up to indicate my state of health. You know, Librach up, sideways, down, you know that kind of thing, so people don't ask the same question. Everyone asks am I well? Well, as well as can be expected" — he took another long draw on his sippy cup — "that doesn't cut it, what is expected? So anyways it's been an interesting few days."

He paused. In one of my previous lives, the one in which I was a journalist, these silences in the middle of an interview could be uncomfortable. I could feel the subject shift in their seat, wonder if perhaps I'd run out of questions, or if they'd simply stymied me. Anxious to present themselves and their story in the best possible light. Conscious always of the scratch of the pen on my notepad, or of the steady hum of the voice recorder. This silence wasn't like that. There was an anxiety embedded in all our conversations because we were both aware of how little time we had, the need to capture as much as we could before Larry's mind blurred and his body shut down forever. But I was in no hurry to move to the next topic, the next thought. He was so obviously weaker today. I let him rest for a moment, gather his resources.

There was what writers call a beat — a moment of time — where nothing really happened, before he exclaimed, "Oh!" and reached for his BlackBerry.

One of the things Larry struggled with was expressing a sense of his spirituality. He wasn't overtly religious, although he brought his children up in the Jewish tradition, and he observed Judaism's high days and holidays (Rosh Hashanah, Yom Kippur, Passover, et cetera). When he was crafting the funeral address for his own funeral he'd been impressed by his rabbi's take on spirituality, but that expressed more about her spirituality and her faith than his own.

"I had an interesting email from my friend Leo Pessini in Brazil. He was the provincio, which is like a bishop for this order of San Camillus in South America. And in the middle of this email he talks about what I'm doing. He says I'm doing something very transcendent and spiritual, just by opening myself up to people to see and understand the process of dying a little better. Here's a Roman Catholic priest who doesn't know what to say. Even he was amazed."

Anyone else might have sounded boastful, but I sensed relief more than pride. One of the final pieces had snapped into place for Larry. It wasn't a profound philosophical insight, but it helped him to see that for him finding meaning and purpose at the end of life was intimately connected with everything he'd done over the past few months. He'd shared his journey with his wife and family. Allowed them to grieve and grieved with them. Sat with me, week after week. Explained to me what it's like to walk this path. So many have walked it before, but here was somebody who understood the issues walking it and seeing things that most others haven't noticed before.

For the first time our talk was punctuated by several phone calls. There had always been phone calls, but today Larry was answering his phone. Russell called to arrange a visit later in the day. He was headed to Israel with his family the following day for a vacation, and he wanted to see Larry before he left. And then Judith, his daughter, called.

"Hello, Darling Daughter. They're open, yes. Tired. Yeah, loaded 45. Yeah, right, okay. And a buxom blond, yeah. Which one's first? I guess I'd better do the buxom blond first, no point the other way around. Okay, bye."

"She's got your sense of humour then."

"Yeah, well, Faye's been asking constantly, what do you need next, what do you need next? Finally last week I said 'a loaded 45.' It took her about a half hour to figure out what that was and then she came back at me. So now when she asks me what I want I say a loaded 45 and she just ignores me totally, of course. But Judith still hasn't gotten the idea [that] she can drop by any time.

"But it's Faye I really worry about. She's really been under a lot of stress as I said, so I need to try to sort that out. She takes it all on, my wife. She thinks she has it under control. She doesn't, and everybody's telling her how tired and awful she looks, which doesn't help her."

Three days later Faye emailed to tell me Larry wanted to give me an update, but he wasn't strong enough to dictate anything into the computer. He dictated a few words to her instead:

"Thoughts for Thursday August 8: Getting weaker. Hard to think straight. This may mean that you will need to add words to all this, not just to increase the verbiage but also to make it more understandable.

"This morning when I woke up I could tell I was even weaker. How is this so? Not clear, but seems to be happening rapidly. Main goal for me is that I last another week so I can see my granddaughters when they return from camp.

"More to come later...."

I called the following day to arrange our next meeting. Faye was hesitant — there was the briefest of pauses on the line — before she passed the phone over to Larry. I asked him if he'd be strong enough to meet again the following week. "I have to be," he said. But his voice was faint, and difficult to understand because of his slur. We arranged to meet the following Monday, and I told him to rest before I rang off.

I called before setting off, as I usually did. I moved slowly that morning, because I had a strong suspicion our meeting wouldn't be happening. I didn't call until around 9:15. The instant Faye answered I could hear something in her voice. There was the tiredness, yes, but it was also flat, without inflection. No up notes at all. The voice of someone who has lost hope.

I didn't ask my usual questions: How was Larry? Was he up for a visit today? I just blurted out something about planning to visit today if he was up to it. "He won't be able to see you today. He's confused, and he's not making any sense most of the time. There wouldn't be any point."

Her son-in-law was driving to camp to fetch their granddaughters. They were due home on Wednesday, but Faye thought Wednesday might be too late. They didn't want to take the risk.

"I don't think Larry will be able to do any more interviews. I hope you have enough for the book." She told me she would let me know if there were any developments.

Funny, I didn't really think of them as interviews. Not toward the end at least. To me they were conversations. Conversations on dying, with an expert on death.

Did I have enough for the book? I imagine I would always want more. But no number of conversations would have alleviated the weight of this news. That I'd probably seen Larry for the last time.

It wouldn't be fair, or true, to say that the news left me numb, although there was a certain unreality to it (expected as it was) that made it feel like numbness. All I knew is I couldn't think, couldn't focus, couldn't work. I should have been working hard, working on the transcriptions, organizing my thoughts around our many discussions, fitting Larry's thoughts into the overall narrative. Blending and refining. But I couldn't focus on that.

Perhaps it was because, after months of meeting and talking, that phase of this journey was now over. That work was now done, and a new phase would begin, in which I'd process and refine, review and research. But I didn't think that was it either. It felt like an end, certainly, but not in that way. It felt as if a certain set of possibilities would die along with Larry. The things he could yet have done. The people he had yet to teach and inspire. Those things would now be lost to us. What is left is this book: his last effort to capture something that could be handed down, to make some sort of difference for patients and the doctors who treat them.

I felt immeasurably sad that I'd lost a friend. That many had lost one of their best friends. But my sadness bled beyond those selfish borders. I was sad Canada had lost Larry. Of course, I knew he was still alive, for the moment. But Faye didn't expect him to live out the week. So that day I said goodbye to my friend Larry.

By Wednesday I'd still had no news from Faye. My thoughts constantly drifted toward him. That day Natalie snuck me into a lunchtime lecture on pancreatic cancer at Mount Sinai, given by Larry's oncologist, Malcolm Moore.

It was another of those instances of self-torture to which I seemed to be prone at the time. It was necessary research, and normally I enjoy this part of the work. I love to uncover those tiny shards of trivia that bring a story to life. But in this particular case those shards were driven straight under my skin, the moment I picked one of them up. During the previous month or so, in addition to *The Emperor of All Maladies*, I'd read Christopher Hitchens's essays for *Vanity Fair* on his esophageal cancer, and at the suggestion of Natalie Onuska, a friend from my critique circle in Toronto, Joan Didion's memoir of loss, grief, and mourning, *The Year of Magical Thinking*. At that point I was reading Julian Barnes's reflections on death, *Nothing to Be Frightened Of*, at the suggestion of Robyn Read. The next on the stack was Stephen Cave's reflections on our species's seemingly irrepressible desire to live forever, *Immortality*, again at Larry's suggestion.

Natalie worried that I needed to give myself time off, that constantly reflecting on death wasn't healthy. In this she had a point. It was definitely not making me more cheerful. But then, would I have been likely to be cheerful anyway, given the circumstances? There's a dopey illogic to this. My misery was not a whit helpful to Larry. But it was hard not to feel I betrayed him whenever I forgot, for a moment, his suffering. It may not have hurt him for us to have enjoyed ourselves during those few months of his dying, but I felt in some difficult to pin down way, it showed a lack of fine feeling. A callousness.

It had been a holiday in Canada on the previous Monday, and after visiting Larry we'd wandered about a bit (me to buy a book on death) before stopping for lunch at a pub. The menu was light on healthy choices, but I was hungry and wasn't inclined to go in search of other more healthy establishments, so I ordered (to Natalie's horror) a club sandwich. This (for me) blasé attitude toward my diet was a feature of those days when I'd been to see Larry. There's no logic that comes close to explaining it. What was I thinking? "Life is short so I may as well make it somewhat shorter?" Perhaps. Seeing Larry was certainly a powerful *memento mori*, and what was the point of all my self-denial when I'd end up just as dead, with or without the bacon? There is the quality-of-life argument, of course. Spending my last years with chronic atherosclerosis doesn't sound like a lot of fun. I always imagined myself coming to a quick end: skiing into a tree at age eighty, or dying in a failed parachute incident at ninety-five.

But the spectacle of Larry provided other possibilities in the panoply of ways to die. Far less alluring ones. And if that is to be my end, I may as well get all of my living (and bacon) in while I still can.

Interesting, however, that this shifted perspective seemed to last a few hours, as if it were a drug whose potency wore off with the passage of a short amount of time. The next day I would be back in the gym, avoiding saturated fats, sugar, and sodium, and munching down quinoa, bulgar wheat, and wild rice.

On Thursday, August 15, Natalie bustled around the kitchen: reached into the fridge to find something for lunch, packed a box of tea bags, made sure she had her iPhone, her keys, her notes. Thursdays were busy days for her at the Centre, the one day of the week when all the Centre's physicians were in the office. She liked to get in early. She was about ready to go when her phone buzzed with an incoming email. Her head drooped to the device. There was a sharp intake of breath, her hand flew to her mouth. Just like in Bequia, when we first got the news about Larry.

She swiped away the lock screen, entered her passcode, and read. Tears pregnant and hot, dime- and nickel-sized, burst on the slate floor. This time I didn't need to speculate while I hugged her.

She didn't say anything. When we unfolded from each other she simply handed me the phone. The email was from Jennifer Arvanitis, the physician who was on call the previous night.

> **Open this in a quiet moment please**
>
> Hello all,
>
> It is with a broken heart that I need to inform you that our dear Larry died peacefully at home around 3:00 this morning, surrounded by his family.
>
> On behalf of the Centre, I just want to thank David and Albert so much for their outstanding care to Larry and his family.
>
> There are no words to describe this monumental loss, obviously.
>
> Kindly continue to support each other, as you have done over the past four months.

CHAPTER 24

Funeral

Jewish custom calls for the body of the deceased to be buried as quickly as possible. Larry was buried the day after he died, on Friday, August 16. Being mid-August, many of his friends and colleagues were on vacation, but despite that the memorial chapel was full to bursting.

There were several eulogies. Larry's son, David, and his son-in-law, Ryan, both spoke. Then Larry's cousin stepped up. I suppose most people expected another eulogy. That's not what they got. Not at all.

What they got was a message from Larry. He'd warned me to expect it, so I knew it was coming. He would have been amused by the frisson of surprise that rippled through the congregation as they realized they were hearing Larry's final words to them.

> Family, friends and colleagues.
>
> You know that I could not resist getting the last word in, in this case quite literally. I know that it is unusual for the person being honoured by the funeral to say a few words, but bear with me for a brief few minutes. The purpose of my remarks is to thank you all for being part of my life, for helping to give my life meaning and for all the support you have shown me and my family over the last few months.
>
> My wife, Faye, has been so much a part of my life that I feel that we were truly beshert, truly meant for each other. The nerdy medical student and the quiet Romanian beauty

were bound to meet up and share so much and produce an incredible life together. Figele, you have been a paragon spouse, mother, bubbie, teacher, friend, principal. I could not have asked for anything more other than to spend more time together. It has been quite a journey together. One of my major regrets is that we did not have more time. Please take good care of yourself and the family. To my family and friends, I challenge you to help Faye grieve well and to continue your friendships and relationships with her in my absence.

> I have said many times over the last few months that my children David and Judith have been absolutely amazing in providing me with support, comfort and love. If my life's meaning can be reflected in anything, it is in the quality persons that both my children have become. They are successful as parents, as spouses, as friends and as children. Not sure what role I played in all this but I can and will take some credit. Judith and David, please continue to be proud of who you are. Cast aside any self-doubts. You have become wonderful parents, friends, colleagues and whole people. You have chosen your spouses, Ryan and Sandra, very wisely and may your love continue to grow and deepen.

> My grandchildren, Ella, Jesse and Finn, were an important part of my life. I want to thank them in particular for making me feel like a very important person indeed. I love you so so much.

> To my sister Barbara, never doubt my love for you. You have always stood by my side and I value your friendship.

> For the rest of you, may your journey through life be as meaningful as mine was. Cherish each day. Make sure your life has balance. Make sure your family always has a place in your hearts but also reach out and carry out your social responsibilities to ensure your fellow man is cared for.

I lowered my head and covered my mouth with my hand. Not that I thought my smile was inappropriate, just that someone seeing it might misinterpret. I smiled because it was so typical of Larry to exhort us beyond the grave to care for each other. During his illness I'd seen him lash out (the closest I ever came to seeing him angry) at those who prey on vulnerable loved ones' false hopes and expectations. The real hope, the hope we can all aspire to and play a part in fulfilling, is that we should care for each other. The healthy for the sick, the strong for the weak, the wealthy for the less well off. Larry embodied this spirit in his life, and he demonstrated it fully in the manner of his death. He was true to himself to the end of his life. Typically, he was true to himself beyond the end of his life. He never let a teachable moment pass. If dying as we have lived is one of the components of a good death, then Larry achieved his goal.

Larry didn't quite get the final word in the event. Rabbi Yael Splansky saved her remarks until last. She catalogued Larry's major achievements, but it was far from a dry list of appointments and awards. She'd grown to know Larry in the previous few months, as I had. It may have been my imagination, but I sensed a tremor in her voice as she read, as if she too had fallen prey to his infuriating charm.

After the service the congregation filed out to the car park. It was a hot, sunny day and we loitered around in our shirtsleeves as we waited for the funeral procession to assemble itself. It was a twenty-minute drive from the memorial chapel to the cemetery. The procession was, I'm guessing, at least a mile long. Long enough at least that the organizers had to hire OPP officers to control the intersections along the route. We turned on our highway brights and four-way flashers and followed toward the end of the line.

Larry was buried in a quiet corner of the cemetery, a maple tree casting its shadow over the plot. He would have liked this spot. It would have reminded him to take a moment, stop, relish life. To listen, as he used to say, "to the waves wave."

ACKNOWLEDGEMENTS

Without Larry's widow, Faye, this book could not have been written. She opened her home to me and allowed me to steal some of Larry's final precious hours. It was an act of astonishing generosity. Larry's daughter, Judith, also gave time to help fill in some gaps and provide background material for scenes where I was not present. Larry's son, David, also provided vital background and context.

My friend and sometime-editor Robyn Read helped shape early versions of John's story and the story of my heart attack, and was a sounding board for me as Larry's story developed. Her artful hand is everywhere to be found in this book.

I took a very early version of chapter 1 to the Banff Centre for the Arts and workshopped it with Charlotte Gill. She provided valuable insights and suggestions, as did my fellow classmates: Susan Boland, Emma Gilchrist, Sarah Pollard, Sheila Meads, Renee Hetherington, Andrea Verwey, and Kaija Pepper.

While I'm thanking colleagues, I should mention Sue Reynolds and James Dewar, who open their home to a few lucky writers twice a year to allow them to write in peace and tranquility. Their feedback, and the feedback of the other writers on the retreat (Deepam Wadds and Trish Boyco) was thoughtful while their enthusiasm for *Conversations on Dying* was inspiring. Finally, I should mention my Toronto critique group Meta4 (Laure Baudot, Phebe Tsang, and Natalie Onuska). Natalie in particular helped me develop some of these scenes from early journal notes.

Kristen den Hartog helped me develop the book proposal. Her timely and sensible advice helped enormously, and was given so generously. When it was ready she put me in touch with her literary agency, where I happened upon the perfect agent for this book: the talented, enthusiastic, and savvy Trena White. The ideal advocate, as it turned out.

Thanks too to Dundurn's Margaret Bryant for believing in the book, and acquiring it for Dundurn. My editor, Cheryl Hawley, provided sensitive, intelligent suggestions that always improved the book.

My twin sister, Sally Compobassi, nudged my memory whenever it failed me, as I tried to reconstruct the scenes of my brother John's final few months. My brothers Stephen and Barry Dwyer also helped me fill in some of the blanks.

Kate Dockrill and Celeste Kiberd (a mother–daughter team) transcribed my recordings of my conversations with Larry, which saved me a huge amount of time. For Kate this was a labour of love: she was Larry's assistant when he was director of the Latner Centre, and knew his voice better than anyone outside his family.

Thanks too for the support and cheerleading of my friends and colleagues at the Writers' Community of Durham County. They are too many to mention each of them by name, but I think particularly of Ruth E. Walker and Jennifer Madore.

Drs. Russell Goldman, Sandy Buchman, and Victor Cellarius all helped to check the book for errors (medical and otherwise). Any that remain are my responsibility.

Were it not for the intervention and care of Dr. Juan Carlos Monge and his team at St. Michael's Hospital I may not have survived to write this story, which makes him, at the very least, an accomplice.

When I was at Banff the distinguished Maori author Witi Ihimaera (*The Whale Rider*) warned me to finish the book quickly, because if I took too long "your wife will divorce you." I don't think my wife, Natalie Parry, ever got close to that, but I do know that she has endured long periods when the book absorbed my entire attention, energy, and intellect. I offer her my grateful thanks for putting up with me far past what Witi set as the furthest point of her endurance.

Finally, thanks are due to the Toronto Arts Council and the Ontario Arts Council for providing the grants that helped me write this book. These organizations are part of the reason Ontario has such a thriving literary scene. They are to be treasured.